W9-CCC-719

LIVER AND PANCREATIC DISEASES MANAGEMENT

ADVANCES IN EXPERIMENTAL MEDICINE AND BIOLOGY

Editorial Board:

NATHAN BACK, *State University of New York at Buffalo*

IRUN R. COHEN, *The Weizmann Institute of Science*

DAVID KRITCHEVSKY, *Wistar Institute*

ABEL LAJTHA, N.S. Kline *Institute for Psychiatric Research*

RODOLFO PAOLETTI, *University of Milan*

A Continuation Order Plan is available for this series. A continuation order will bring delivery of each new volume immediately upon publication. Volumes are billed only upon actual shipment. For further information please contact the publisher.

LIVER AND PANCREATIC DISEASES MANAGEMENT

Edited by

Nagy A. Habib and Ruben Canelo

Imperial College School of Medicine, Hammersmith Hospital,
London, United Kingdom

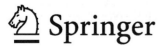 Springer

A C.I.P. Catalogue record for this book is available from the Library of Congress.

ISBN-10 0-387-28548-2 (HB)
ISBN-13 978-0-387-28548-1 (HB)
ISBN-10 0-387-29512-7 (e-book)
ISBN-13 978-0-387-29512-1 (e-book)

Published by Springer,
P.O. Box 17, 3300 AA Dordrecht, The Netherlands.

www.springer.com

Printed on acid-free paper

All rights reserved
© 2006 Springer
No part of this work may be reproduced, stored in a retrieval system, or transmitted
in any form or by any means, electronic, mechanical, photocopying, microfilming,
recording or otherwise, without written permission from the Publisher, with the
exception of any material supplied specifically for the purpose of being entered
and executed on a computer system, for exclusive use by the purchaser of the work.

Printed in the Netherlands.

Preface

The aim of this book is to present a unique compilation of lectures given by international speakers at the Hammersmith Hospital during the Meetings in Hepato-Pancreato-Biliary Surgery and Transplantation 2003–2004. Their experience in the management of patients with liver, bile duct, and pancreas diseases, which is so important to assess the degree of disturbance and to diagnose the causative insult is accurately presented in this edition. New therapeutic approaches, advances in oncology, and diagnostic imaging, which reduce the need for invasive techniques and reach an improvement in survival and quality of life in cancer, is considered. The topic liver pathology is focused first in the management of common bile duct stones in the era of laparoscopic surgery followed by the treatment of primary and secondary liver tumors. Moreover, other attractive topics including advances in the technique of liver resection using radio frequency ablation to minimize the perioperative blood loss is exposed in this edition. New techniques in transplantation of the liver and developments in whole pancreas and pancreatic islet cell transplantation is accurately analyzed. Modern literature has been reviewed with special reference to articles of general interest. We are indebted to many colleges for their generous contribution to this edition, who writing by individual experience in their field provided for this volume an invaluable insight into this difficult area. We hope that this edition will be an up-to-dated account of diseases of the liver, biliary tract, and pancreas, including transplantation of value for surgeons, physicians, and pathologists and also a reference book for medical students.

Contents

Isolated Hepatic Perfusion: Treating Unresectable Liver Metastases

JEFFREY M. FARMA, JAMES F. PINGPANK, and
H. RICHARD ALEXANDER
Surgical Metabolism Section, Surgery Branch, National Cancer Institute, CRC, Rm. 4W-5952,
10 Center Drive, MSC 1201, Bethesda, MD 20892-1201, USA

1. INTRODUCTION

Patients with metastatic carcinoma to the liver have a dismal prognosis. Numerous types of cancer have a predilection to metastasize predominantly or exclusively to the liver including colorectal cancer, ocular melanoma, cholangiocarcinoma, and neuroendocrine neoplasms. In the United States, approximately 145,000 new cases of colorectal cancer will be diagnosed in 2005. Of these patients, 20% will have metastatic disease at the time of diagnosis, predominately involving the liver.[1] In select patients, surgical resection performed with curative intent remains the standard of care. A recent review of 1,001 patients undergoing liver resection for metastatic colorectal cancer demonstrated 5- and 10-year survival rates of 37 and 22%, respectively.[2] In patients with unresectable metastatic colorectal cancer, median survival after treatment with aggressive systemic chemotherapy ranges from 11 to 20 months.[3–5] If untreated, median survival is 6–12 months following the natural course of the disease.[6]

In patients with ocular melanoma, 63% of patients have metastatic disease at the time of death, with initial metastases in the liver present in 70–93% of patients.[7–10] Metastasis occurs hematogenously from the eye, with the liver being the sole site in approximately 80% of patients.[11–13] Metastatic neuroendocrine neoplasms tend to be more indolent; however, patients are often symptomatic from unopposed production of peptide hormones resulting in significant morbidity.[14]

Various strategies have emerged to treat primary or metastatic hepatic neoplasms. Of these strategies, the most important is surgical resection; unfortunately, the majority of metastatic disease to the liver is unresectable at the time of diagnosis. Modalities used to control unresectable liver disease include systemic chemotherapy, local ablative therapy, embolization, and regional infusion therapy. Local ablative therapies include radiofrequency ablation alone or in combination with resection, cryotherapy, or ethanol injection. Embolization has been utilized in attempts to limit blood flow and nutrients to the tumor and can be performed with or without the addition of directed intra-arterial chemotherapy.

The liver is a unique organ allowing complete isolation of its vascular supply to deliver directed regional therapy. Studies have demonstrated that liver metastases recruit their blood supply predominantly from the hepatic artery rather than the portal vein.[15,16] This unique vascularity provides an opportunity to deliver higher concentrations of chemotherapy

1

N. A. Habib and R. Canelo (eds.), Liver and Pancreatic Diseases Management, 1–16.
© 2006 *Springer. Printed in The Netherlands.*

directly to the liver metastases while largely sparing normal hepatic parenchyma. Infusion treatments that have been explored include hepatic artery infusion (HAI) using an implanted pump, HAI with hemofiltration, chemoembolization, selective internal radiation, and isolated hepatic perfusion (IHP). This review will concentrate on the development and outcomes of the IHP procedure.

Ausman reported the first clinical IHP performed in 1961.[17] Interest was limited secondary to the high morbidity of the procedure and limited data supporting its efficacy. As publications demonstrating the dramatic anti-tumor effects of tumor necrosis factor (TNF), interferon-γ, and melphalan in isolated limb perfusion for extremity sarcoma and in-transit melanoma surfaced, renewed interest in IHP using these agents emerged.[18-20] The IHP procedure allows complete isolation of the liver from the systemic circulation using an extracorporeal circuit consisting of a roller pump, reservoir, heat exchanger, and oxygenator. Once the liver is placed on the circuit, high doses of therapeutic agents can be delivered at levels that would normally be limited by systemic toxicities. In addition, regional hyperthermia can be administered enhancing vascular permeability and allowing increased selective delivery of the therapeutic agent.[21] There are limited systemic toxicities. Some agents that have been studied in clinical trials include 5-fluorouracil, mitomycin C (MMC), melphalan, and TNF.

2.   SURGICAL TECHNIQUE

The surgical technique of IHP has been previously described in the literature.[22] All patients undergo a preoperative computed tomography of the chest, abdomen, and pelvis, as well as magnetic resonance imaging of the liver to fully evaluate the degree of hepatic disease and define the hepatic vasculature. Preoperative lab work includes hematologic, chemistry, liver, and coagulation profiles.

Initial abdominal exploration is performed through a limited right subcostal incision. The liver, porta hepatis, and peritoneal cavity are examined for extent of disease and to rule out evidence of disseminated intra-abdominal disease. The procedure is aborted if extensive lymphadenopathy outside of the porta hepatis or peritoneal implants are discovered. Periportal lymphadenopathy is resected prior to perfusion and does not portend perfusion. Once the decision is made to proceed, the subcostal incision is extended and the liver is completely mobilized along with the retrohepatic inferior vena cava (IVC). All venous tributaries to the IVC are ligated from the renal veins to the diaphragm including the right adrenal vein and the phrenic veins. The porta hepatis is dissected and skeletonized. Any periportal lymph nodes are dissected and removed at this time. A cholecystectomy is performed to prevent chemical induced cholecystitis.

Incisions are made in the left or right axilla and the left or right groin to identify the axillary and saphenous veins for placement of the venous cannulae (Fig. 1). A veno-venous bypass circuit is set up channeling blood from the IVC via the saphenous vein catheter into the systemic circulation via the axillary vein. Initially, portal blood flow was incorporated into this circuit; however, our current technique is to occlude the portal vein with a vascular clamp prior to perfusion.

Next, a segment of the infrahepatic IVC is isolated between vascular clamps, and a venous return cannula is positioned so that the tip is just below the hepatic veins. This

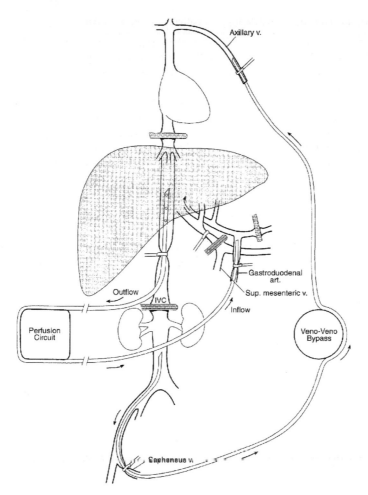

Figure 1. Illustration of IHP circuit. Schema of the IHP circuit illustrating vascular isolation of the liver. Therapeutic agents are administered via the gastroduodenal artery into the hepatic arterial system. Blood from the infrahepatic vena cava is shunted to the systemic circulation using a veno-venous bypass circuit. Vascular occluding clamps are depicted on the suprarenal and subdiaphragmatic IVC, the hepatic artery, and the portal vein.

cannula is used as an outflow draining venous effluent. An arterial inflow cannula is placed into the gastroduodenal artery and positioned so that both the right and left hepatic arteries are perfused equally. If anomalous anatomy exists, dual arterial inflow cannulas are utilized. Vascular clamps are then placed across the suprahepatic IVC just below the diaphragm, the proximal common hepatic artery, and the portal vein.

Adequate hyperthermia is monitored throughout the procedure with hepatic temperature probes. Perfusion parameters from 51 patients treated with IHP are listed in Table 1.[23] Stable parameters are reached quickly at the outset of the perfusion. In our initial experience, we routinely monitored for perfusate leak (Fig. 2); this has been abandoned due to such a low

Table 1. Perfusion and operative data from 51 patients treated with IHP

Melphalan dose (mg) 1.5 mg/kg	106 (75–140)
Perfusion flow rate (ml/min)	831 (600—1,050)
Arterial line pressure (mmHg)	165 (103–225)
Veno-venous bypass flow rate (l/min)	1.8 (1.2–2.4)
Central liver temperature (°C)	39.9 (39–40.6)
Operative time (h)	8.5 (6.3–12)
Estimated blood loss (l)	2.2 (1–5)
Duration of perfusion (min)	60
Perfusate composition	700 ml crystalloid; 300 ml Packed RBCs; 2,000 U heparin; 45 ± 15 mEq. NaHCO$_3$
Post-perfusion hepatic artery flush	1.5 l crystalloid; 1.5 l colloid

rate of systemic leak. Once the perfusion is complete, the liver is flushed to remove any of the residual chemotherapy or biological therapy used. The vessels are de-cannulated and venotomies are primarily closed. Overall treatment related mortality in recently reported series of patients treated with IHP is <5%.[24]

3. OVERVIEW OF CLINICAL TRIALS OF IHP

A few institutions have published reports detailing their single center experience using IHP (Table 2). Marinelli et al. described their results using normothermic IHP with MMC or melphalan in patients with metastatic colorectal cancer confined to the liver. Of the initial nine patients treated with MMC, two had a complete remission with a median survival of 17 months; however, four of these patients had hepatic veno-occlusive disease. Due to the high morbidity associated with MMC, they began to use melphalan in the perfusion circuit and treated 24 patients with an escalating dose of melphalan and 26 patients with 200 mg melphalan.

Our initial experience in the Surgery Branch at the National Cancer Institute with IHP has focused on phase I or II trials utilizing melphalan with and without the addition of TNF (Table 3). In our initial phase I trial, we studied escalating doses of TNF alone administered during IHP. The maximum tolerated dose (MTD) of TNF was demonstrated to be 1.5 mg with a dose-limiting toxicity (DLT) being coagulopathy. The following phase I trial, evaluated the combination of melphalan and TNF administered during IHP. In this dose escalation study, the MTD of melphalan was 1.5 mg/kg and TNF was 1.0 mg. The DLT with the combination of melphalan and TNF was hepatic veno-occlusive disease.[25] We have shown that TNF in the perfusate is associated with additional systemic toxicities compared to melphalan alone. This may be due to the effect of TNF on hepatic cytokine synthesis with increased levels of inflammatory mediators, such as interleukin 6 and interleukin 8, in the perfusate during IHP and transient systemic levels immediately after. All of these associated toxicities were transient, reversible, and easy to treat.[26]

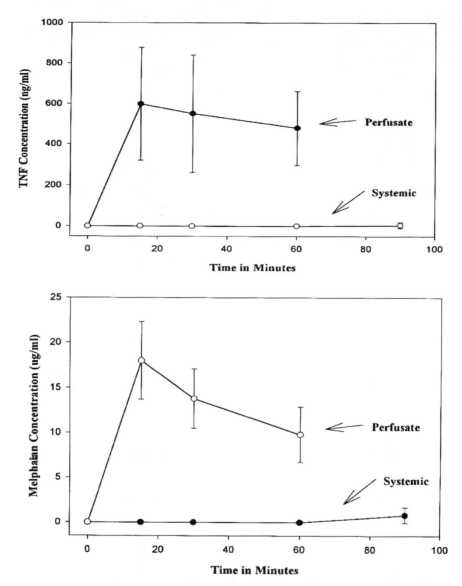

Figure 2. Pharmacokinetics of TNF and melphalan during IHP. The plots represent mean (±standard deviation) of TNF concentration (upper panel) and melphalan concentration (lower panel) over time in the systemic circulation and the perfusate in 32 patients treated with IHP.

4.   METASTATIC COLORECTAL CANCER

The largest clinical trials of IHP have evaluated patients with metastatic colorectal cancer to the liver. In one study, patients with metastatic colorectal cancer to the liver were

Table 2. Summary of large series of IHP reported after 1998

Author	N	Agent(s)	Dose(s)	Histology	Temperature (°C)	Response rate (%)	CR[a] (%)	PR[b] (%)	Median survival (months)
Marinelli et al. (1998).[43]	9	MMC[c]	30 mg/m²	Colorectal	37	–	22	–	17
	50	Melphalan	0.5–4 mg/kg or 200 mg		37	12	2	10	–
Alexander et al. (1998).[44]	34	Melphalan/TNF[d]	1.5 mg/kg, 1.0 mg	Mixed	39.5–40	75	3	72	9 (mean)
Vahrmeijer et al. (2000).[45]	24	Melphalan	0.5–4.0 mg/kg	Colorectal	37–38	29	4	17	19
Alexander et al. (2000).[30]	11	Melphalan	1.5–2.5 mg/kg	Ocular melanoma	39.5–40	62	9.5	52	9
	11	Melphalan/TNF	1.5–2.5 mg/kg, 1 mg						
Libutti et al. (2000).[22]	50	Melphalan/TNF	1.5 mg/kg, 1 mg	Mixed	39–40	75	2	73	–
Bartlett et al. (2001).[23]	32	Melphalan/TNF	1.5 mg/kg, 1 mg	Colorectal	39–40	76	–	77	16
	19	Melphalan/FUDR[e]/ LV[f]	1.5 mg/kg, 0.2 mg/kg/day 15 mg/m²/day				–	74	27
Alexander et al. (2003).[31]	29	Melphalan	1.5 mg/kg	Ocular melanoma	39–40	62	10	52	12.1
Rothbarth et al. (2003).[27]	73	Melphalan	200 mg	Colorectal	39.5	59	4	55	29

a Complete response.
b Partial response.
c Mitomycin C.
d Tumor necrosis factor.
e Floxuridine.
f Leucovorin.

Table 3. NCI Surgery Branch experience with IHP

Trial type	Trial description	Patient number/ dates of accrual	Results
Phase I	Escalating dose of TNF[a]	17 (6/93–6/94)	DLT[b] coagulopathy MTD[c] TNF = 1.5 mg
Phase I	Escalating dose of TNF and melphalan	14 (7/94–11/95)	DLT VOD[d] melphalan + TNF MDT: 1.0 mg TNF/1.5 mg/kg melphalan
Phase II	Melphalan/TNF	54 (12/95–8/97)	RR: 75%
Phase II	Melplalan/TNF + HAI[e] with FUDR[f] for metastatic colorectal cancer	9 (2/97–7/97)	RR: 75%
Phase I	Escalating dose of melphalan	45 (9/97–6/99)	PV/HA[g] IHP-DLT ascites HA IHP-DLT VOD MTD: 1.5 mg/kg melphalan
Phase II	Melphalan alone	81 (6/99–5/04)	Completing accrual
Phase III	IV/HAI chemotherapy for colorectal cancer	18 (7/02–6/03)	Closed, equivalence
Phase II	Melphalan alone for colorectal cancer as a second-line therapy	1 (8/04–current)	Accruing

[a] Tumor necrosis factor.
[b] Dose-limiting toxicity.
[c] Maximum tolerated dose.
[d] Veno-occlusive disease.
[e] Hepatic artery infusion.
[f] Floxuridine.
[g] Portal vein/hepatic artery.

treated on a trial combining IHP with melphalan (1.5 mg/kg) with or without TNF (1 mg) with post-operative continuous HAI of FUDR (0.2 mg/kg/day) and leucovorin (15 mg/m^2/day). The HAI regimen was initiated 6 weeks after recovery from IHP and included 14 days of HAI, repeated every 28 days for up to 12 cycles. In 2001, the results of 51 patients treated on this study were published; 32 patients received IHP with melphalan and TNF and 19 patients received melphalan alone followed by post-operative HAI. Approximately 50% of the patients had failed previous treatment for metastatic colorectal cancer and had advanced hepatic disease. There was one peri-operative death (2%). There were significant grade 3/4 toxicities associated with the treatment. Transient hypotension and hyperbilirubinemia were more common in the group receiving TNF. Twenty-four of 31 patients who had IHP alone had a partial response (77%); the median duration of response for IHP alone was 8.5 months with a median overall survival of 16 months (Fig. 3). In the group treated with IHP followed by HAI therapy, 14 of 19 patients had a partial response (74%); the median duration of response in this group was 14.5 months with a median overall survival of 27 months.[23]

Rothbarth et al. recently published their series of 73 patients enrolled on a phase II study using IHP with melphalan to treat metastatic colorectal cancer to the liver. Seventy-one

Pre-IHP

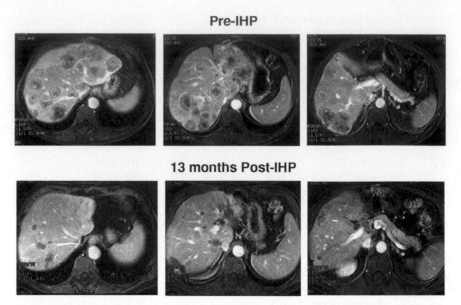

13 months Post-IHP

Figure 3. T1-weighted magnetic resonance imaging studies in a patient with unresectable colorectal metastases to the liver. This patient was treated with a 60-min hyperthermic IHP with melphalan alone. The upper panel shows extensive disease prior to treatment. The lower panel shows corresponding images taken 13 months post-treatment with IHP demonstrating a stable partial response.

patients were perfused with melphalan (200 mg) via the hepatic artery and portal vein ($n = 64$) or the portal vein alone ($n = 7$). Their operative mortality was 5.6%. In their patients, 16% had grade 3–4 hepatotoxicity 1 week after IHP which was transient. Overall response rate was 59%, with three patients having a complete response. Median time to progression was 7.7 months with an overall median survival of 28.8 months.[27]

Individuals who experience disease progression confined to the liver after first-line systemic chemotherapy regimens have limited response with second- and third-line chemotherapy strategies. For example, patients who have had tumor progression on an irinotecan, 5FU, and leucovorin (IFL) regimen and undergo second-line treatment with an oxaliplatin-based (FOLFOX4) regimen, had an objective response rate of only 9.9%, with a median time to progression of 4.6 months.[3] We recently analyzed the efficacy of IHP in patients with progressive metastatic colorectal disease of the liver after treatment with irinotecan-based chemotherapy. Between 1993 and 2003, 25 patients were identified who were treated using IHP with melphalan (1.5 mg/kg) after having progressive disease after irinotecan. There was 1 complete response (4%) and 14 partial responses (56%), with a median duration of 12 months (Table 4). Thirteen patients progressed systemically at a median of 5 months. Median overall survival was 12 months and 2-year survival was 28% (Fig. 4). These data support the continued clinical evaluation of IHP as a second-line therapy for patients with metastatic colorectal cancer confined to the liver, who have failed irinotecan-based chemotherapy regimens.[28]

Table 4. Results of treatment in 25 patients with metastatic colorectal cancer isolated to the liver treated with IHP after progression on irinotecan-based chemotherapy regimen

Group	n	Radiographic response	Mean duration (months)
Overall	25	15 (60%)	13.2 (5–35)
IHP alone	13	7 (54%)	8.6 (5–13)
IHP + HAI[a]	12	8 (67%)	17.3 (11–35)

[a] Hepatic artery infusion.

5. METASTATIC OCULAR MELANOMA

Ocular melanoma has a predilection to metastasize to the liver. Metastatic ocular melanoma has proven to be resistant to most systemically administered chemotherapy and immunotherapy regimens.[29] We have conducted both phase I and II trials and reported the results using IHP with melphalan with and without the addition of TNF to treat patients with ocular melanoma metastatic to the liver. Initial results of 22 patients treated with IHP with melphalan with or without TNF demonstrated an overall response rate of 62%. Two patients achieved a complete response and 11 patients had a partial response. Median duration of hepatic response was 9 months with two patients surviving greater than 3 years after treatment.[30]

In 2003, we published an updated and larger series using IHP with melphalan alone to treat patients with metastatic ocular melanoma to the liver. Twenty-nine patients were treated with a 60-min IHP using 1.5 mg/kg melphalan. There were three (10%) patients who achieved a complete response (Fig. 5). Fifteen patients (52%) had a partial response with a mean duration of 10 months, for an overall response rate of (62%) (Table 5). At a median follow-up of 30.7 months, the median actuarial progression-free and overall survivals were 8 and 12.1 months, respectively (Fig. 6). The liver was the site of initial progression in 17 of the 25 patients who recurred. A Cox model analysis of these patients demonstrated that baseline LDH $\leq$ 160 was a highly significant independent prognostic factor for response and survival.[31]

Noter et al. recently published their experience using IHP with high dose melphalan to treat ocular melanoma metastases to the liver. Eight patients were treated by IHP with a 60-min perfusion with melphalan (200 mg). There were no complete responders. Four of the eight patients (50%) had partial response, with two patients having stable disease. Median time to progression was 6.7 months. The overall median survival was 6.7 months, with a 1-year survival of 50% and a 2-year survival of 37.5%.[32]

Other institutions have treated similar patients with ocular melanoma to the liver with various other regional strategies. Using chemoembolization with cisplatin, Mavligit et al. reported an objective response rate of 50% with an overall survival of 1 year.[33] Leyvraz et al. reported a 40% response rate in 31 patients treated with intra-arterial fotemustine (100 mg/m^2) with an 11 month median duration of response and a 14 month overall survival.[34]

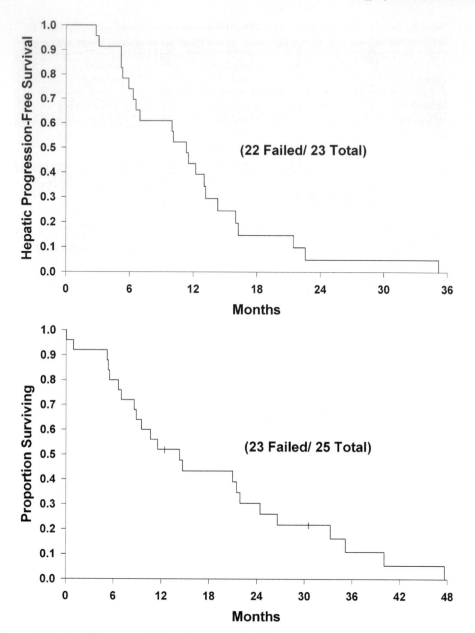

Figure 4. Kaplan–Meier actuarial hepatic progression-free (upper panel) and overall survival (lower panel) in 25 patients treated with IHP for metastatic colorectal cancer to the liver after treatment with irinotecan-based systemic chemotherapy.

Pre-IHP

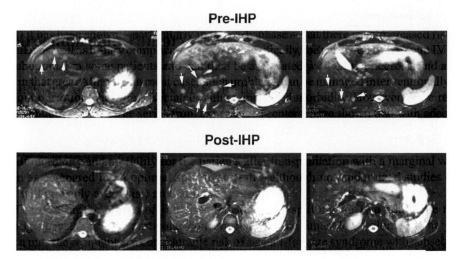

Post-IHP

Figure 5. T2-weighted magnetic resonance imaging studies demonstrating a complete response in a patient with metastatic ocular melanoma to the liver prior to treatment with IHP (upper panel) and 1 year after treatment (lower panel).

6.   PRIMARY HEPATIC NEOPLASMS

In 2005, there will be an estimated 17,500 new cases of primary hepatic and intrahepatic bile duct cancers in the United States, with 15,420 estimated new deaths per year.[1] World-wide, the incidence and mortality of primary hepatic cancer is much greater. In Asia, liver cancer is the most common cause of cancer death in men. Surgical resection is the treatment

Table 5. Results of treatment in 29 patients undergoing IHP for liver metastases from ocular melanoma

	n	%	Duration (months)
Response			
Overall	18	62	
Partial	15	52	10 (5–22)
Complete	3	10	12, 14+[a], 15
Follow-up status[b]			
AWD	10	34	
DOD	19	66	
Follow-up time			
Median			11
Mean			13.5
Range			3–40

[a] "+" signifies ongoing response or stabilization of disease.
[b] AWD, alive with disease; DOD, dead of disease.

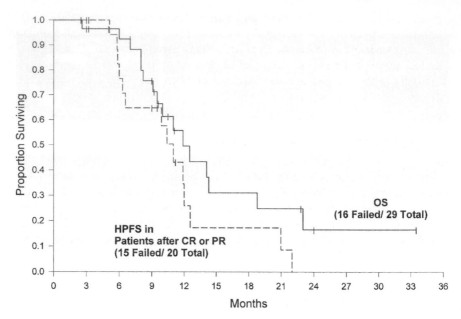

Figure 6. Kaplan–Meier actuarial HPFS in patients with metastatic ocular melanoma to the liver who had either a complete response or partial response after IHP, and overall survival (OS) in 29 patients treated with IHP.

of choice with a 5-year survival rate which approaches 50%; however, only 9–27% of patients will have resectable disease at the time of diagnosis based on tumor location, size, number of lesions, and hepatic reserve.[35,36] Regional therapy although feasible, is often limited by concomitant hepatic cirrhosis, leaving few treatment options available.

We have treated nine patients with unresectable primary hepatic neoplasms with IHP. Five patients had hepatocellular carcinoma and four patients had cholangiocarcinoma or adenocarcinoma of unknown primary origin. IHP was performed with melphalan (1.5 mg/kg) and TNF (1 mg) ($n = 3$) or with melphalan (1.5 mg/kg) alone ($n = 6$). Six of the nine patients (67%) had a partial response to IHP. Mean time to progression was 7.7 months for those who responded to IHP. In patients who responded, overall survival was 16.3 months.[37]

There are few reports in the literature of IHP for primary hepatic neoplasm. Hafström et al. reported four patients with hepatocellular cancer who were treated by IHP with melphalan with or without cisplatin. There were no complete responders, one patient had a partial response, and two patients had stable disease.[38]

7.   METASTATIC NEUROENDOCRINE TUMORS

There are few series describing the treatment of neuroendocrine neoplasms metastatic to the liver by IHP. We recently reported our experience in 13 patients treated by IHP with gastric and pancreatic neuroendocrine cancers. Patients were treated with a one-hour perfusion with melphalan (1.5 or 2.0 mg/kg) and/or TNF (1.0 mg). An overall radiographic response was seen in 50% of patients, all of which had a partial response. An additional four patients had a marginal response. The median hepatic progression-free survival (HPFS) was 7 months, with a median actuarial survival of 48 months. There was one treatment mortality.[39]

8.   METASTATIC SARCOMA

Although there are reports in the literature of dominant hepatic metastases from disseminated sarcoma treated with IHP, most studies have small numbers. Generally, there is extrahepatic disease, in addition to the hepatic metastases, limiting the utility of regional liver perfusion. Hafström et al. treated four patients with leiomyosarcoma by IHP with TNF (40 or 100 μg) and melphalan (0.5 mg/kg) at 39°C. Two patients had a partial response, and the two other patients had stable disease.[40,41]

9.   FUTURE DIRECTIONS

The optimal treatment strategy for patients with metastatic disease to the liver remains a clinical dilemma. We have demonstrated the benefit of IHP as a second-line treatment in patients with metastatic colorectal cancer who have progressed in the setting of irinotecan-based systemic chemotherapy. In the future, we hope to further elucidate the role of IHP as a second-line treatment after oxaliplatin therapy; our institution is developing phase II trials to address this question. In addition, we hope to determine the efficacy of IHP used as a first-line agent in patients with advanced metastatic colorectal cancer to the liver with a significant hepatic burden of disease (>40%).

Recently, we finished a phase I dose escalation and feasibility trial studying a percutaneous hepatic perfusion (PHP) technique using melphalan (Fig. 7).[42] Melphalan is administered selectively to the liver via a percutaneously placed catheter positioned in the proper hepatic artery. A double-balloon catheter is placed in the retrohepatic vena cava to isolate the venous drainage of the liver. Venous effluent is pumped through an extracorporeal bypass circuit, passed through two activated charcoal filters to extract the melphalan and returned to the systemic circulation. This approach offers the benefit of providing multiple treatments, with minimal systemic toxicity without the morbidity associated with an operative procedure. A phase II trial studying PHP in patients with dominant hepatic disease from colorectal cancer, melanoma, and neuroendocrine tumors, has recently started accruing patients.

Most trials have evaluated the use of melphalan in the IHP circuit; however, newer chemotherapeutic or biological agents warrant investigation and could easily be studied using this technique. Although IHP is a technically challenging procedure, we hope to expand its use to other academic centers and have ongoing trials to further evaluate its role in the treatment of unresectable metastatic disease to the liver.

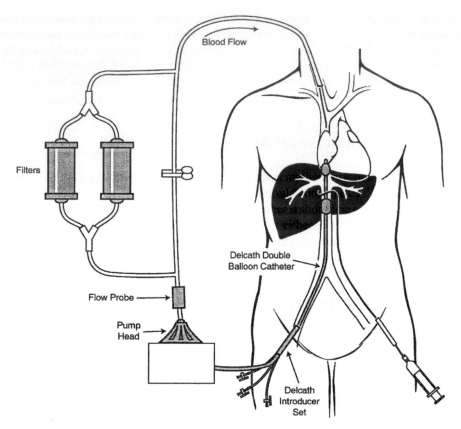

Figure 7. Illustration of PHP circuit using double-balloon catheter. Melphalan is administered directly into the hepatic artery through an infusion catheter placed percutaneously via the femoral artery. Hepatic venous outflow is isolated via a double-balloon catheter in the retrohepatic IVC. Blood is drawn out of the retrohepatic IVC through multiple fenestrations located along the length of the catheter between the cranial and caudal balloons. The blood is then pumped through a pair of activated charcoal filters prior to return to the systemic circulation via an internal jugular vein catheter.

REFERENCES

1. Jemal A, Murray T, Ward E, Samuels A, Tiwari RC, Ghafoor A, Feuer EJ, Thun MJ. Cancer statistics, 2005. *CA Cancer J Clin.* 2005;55:10–30.
2. Fong Y, Fortner J, Sun RL, Brennan MF, Blumgart LH. Clinical score for predicting recurrence after hepatic resection for metastatic colorectal cancer. *Ann Surg.* 1999;230:309–321.
3. Rothenberg MC, Oza AM, Bigelow RH, Berlin JD, Marshall JL, Ramanathan RK, Hart LL, Gupta S, Garay CA, Burger BG, Le Bail N, Haller DG. Superiority of oxaliplatin and fluourouracil–leucovorin compared with either therapy alone in patients with progressive colorectal cancer after irinotecan and fluorouracil–leucovorin: interim results of a phase III trial. *J Clin Oncol.* 2003;21:2059–2069.
4. Hurwitz H, Fehrenbacher L, Novotny W, Cartwright T, Hainsworth J, Heim W, Berlin J, Baron A, Griffing S, Holmgren E, Ferrara N, Fyfe G, Rogers B, Ross R, Kabbinavar F. Bevacizumab plus irinotecan, fluorouracil, and leucovorin for metastatic colorectal cancer. *N Engl J Med.* 2004;350:2335–2342.

5. Saltz LB, Cox JV, Blanke C, Rosen LS, Fehrenbacher L, Moore MJ, Maroun JA, Ackland SP, Locker PK, Pirotta N, Elfring GL, Miller LL. Irinotecan plus fluorouracil and leucovorin for metastatic colorectal cancer. *N Engl J Med.* 2000;343:905–914.
6. Bengmark S, Hafström L. The natural history of primary and secondary malignant tumors of the liver. I. The prognosis for patients with hepatic metastases from colonic and rectal carcinoma by laparotomy. *Cancer.* 1969;23:198–202.
7. Egan KM, Seddon JM, Glynn RJ, Gragoudas ES, Albert DM. Epidemiologic aspects of uveal melanoma. *Surv Ophthalmol.* 1988;32:239–251.
8. Gragoudas ES, Egan KM, Seddon JM, Glynn RJ, Walsh SM, Finn SM, Munzenrider JE, Spar MD. Survival of patients with metastases from uveal melanoma. *Ophthalmology.* 1991;98:383–390.
9. Kath R, Hayungs J, Bornfeld N, Sauerwein W, Höffken K, Seeber S. Prognosis and treatment of disseminated uveal melanoma. *Cancer.* 1993;72:2219–2223.
10. Seregard S, Kock E. Prognostic indicators following enucleation for posterior uveal melanoma. *Acta Opthalmol Scand.* 1995;73:340–344.
11. Tuomaala S, Eskelin S, Tarkkanen A, Kivela T. Population-based assessment of clinical characteristics predicting outcome of conjunctival melanoma in whites. *Invest Ophthalmol Vis Sci.* 2002;43:3399–3408.
12. Shields CL. Conjunctival melanoma: risk factors for recurrence, exenteration, metastasis, and death in 150 consecutive patients. *Trans Am Ophthalmol Soc.* 2000;98:471–492.
13. Rajpal S, Moore R, Karakousis CP. Survival in metastatic ocular melanoma. *Cancer.* 1983;52:334–336.
14. Choti MA, Bulkley GB. Management of hepatic metastases. *Liver Transplant Surg.* 1999;5:65–80.
15. Breedis C, Young G. Blood supply of neoplasms of the liver. *Am J Pathol.* 1954;30:969–985.
16. Lin G, Lunderquist A, Hägerstrand I, Boijsen E. Postmortem examination of the blood supply and vascular pattern of small liver metastases in man. *Surgery.* 1984;96:517–526.
17. Ausman RK. Development of a technic for isolated perfusion of the liver. *N Y State J Med.* 1961;61:3393–3397.
18. Lienard D, Ewalenko P, Delmotti JJ, Renard N, Lejeune FJ. High-dose recombinant tumor necrosis factor alpha in combination with interferon gamma and melphalan in isolation perfusion of the limbs for melanoma and sarcoma. *J Clin Oncol.* 1992;10:52–60.
19. Eggermont AMM, Koops HS, Klausner JM, Kroon BBR, Schlag PM, Liénard D, van Geel AN, Hoekstra HJ, Meller I, Nieweg OE, Kettelhack C, Ben-Ari G, Pector J-C, Lejeune FJ. Isolated limb perfusion with tumor necrosis factor and melphalan for limb salvage in 186 patients with locally advanced soft tissue extremity sarcomas. *Ann Surg.* 1996;224:756–765.
20. Lienard D, Eggermont AM, Schraffordt-Koops H, Kroon BB, Roisenkaimer F, Autier P, Lejeune FJ. Isolated perfusion of the limb with high-dose tumor necrosis factor, interferon gamma and melphalan for melanoma stage III. Results of a multicentre pilot study. *Melanoma Res.* 1994;4:21–26.
21. di Filippo F, Anza M, Rossi CR, Cavaliere F, Botti C, Lise M, Garinei R, Giannarelli D, Vasselli S, Zupi G, Cavaliere R. The application of hyperthermia in regional chemotherapy. *Semin Surg Oncol.* 1998;14:215–223.
22. Libutti SK, Bartlett DL, Fraker DL, Alexander HR. Technique and results of hyperthermic isolated hepatic perfusion with tumor necrosis factor and melphalan for the treatment of unresectable hepatic malignancies. *J Am Coll Surg.* 2000;191:519–530.
23. Bartlett DL, Libutti SK, Figg WD, Fraker DL, Alexander HR. Isolated hepatic perfusion for unresectable hepatic metastases from colorectal cancer. *Surgery.* 2001;129:176–187.
24. Alexander HR Jr, Bartlett DL, Libutti SK. Current status of isolated hepatic perfusion with or without tumor necrosis factor for the treatment of unresectable cancers confined to liver. *Oncologist.* 2000;5:416–424.
25. Alexander HR, Bartlett DL, Libutti SK. Isolated hepatic perfusion: a potentially effective treatment for patients with metastatic or primary cancers confined to the liver. *Cancer J Sci Am.* 1998;4:2–11.
26. Lans TE, Bartlett DL, Libutti SK, Gnant MFX, Liewehr DJ, Venzon DJ, Turner EM, Alexander HR Jr. Role of tumor necrosis factor (TNF) on toxicity and cytokine production following isolated hepatic perfusion (IHP). *Clin Cancer Res.* 2001;7:784–790.
27. Rothbarth J, Pijl ME, Vahrmeijer AL, Hartgrink HH, Tijl FG, Kuppen PJ, Tollenaar RA, van de Velde CJ. Isolated hepatic perfusion with high-dose melphalan for the treatment of colorectal metastasis confined to the liver. *Br J Surg.* 2003;90:1391–1397.
28. Alexander HR Jr, Libutti SK, Pingpank JF, Bartlett DL, Helsabeck C, Beresnev T. Isolated hepatic prefusion for the treatment of patients with colorectal cancer (CRC) liver metastases after irinotecan-based therapy. *Ann Surg Oncol.* 2005 Feb;12(2):138–144.

29. Pyrhonen S, Hahka-Kemppinen M, Muhonen T, Nikkanen V, Eskelin S, Summanen P, Tarkkanen A, Kivela T. Chemoimmunotherapy with bleomycin, vincristine, lomustine, dacarbazine (BOLD), and human leukocyte interferon for metastatic uveal melanoma. *Cancer*. 2002;95:2366–2372.
30. Alexander HR, Libutti SK, Bartlett DL, Puhlmann M, Fraker DL, Bachenheimer LC. A phase I–II study of isolated hepatic perfusion using melphalan with or without tumor necrosis factor for patients with ocular melanoma metastatic to liver. *Clin Cancer Res*. 2000;6:3062–3070.
31. Alexander HR, Libutti SK, Pingpank JF, Steinberg SM, Bartlett DL, Helsabeck C, Beresnev T. Hyperthermic isolated hepatic perfusion (IHP) using melphalan for patients with ocular melanoma metastatic to liver. *Clin Cancer Res*. 2003;9:6343–6349.
32. Noter SL, Rothbarth J, Pijl ME, Keunen JE, Hartgrink HH, Tijl FG, Kuppen PJ, van de Velde CJ, Tollenaar RA. Isolated hepatic perfusion with high-dose melphalan for the treatment of uveal melanoma metastases confined to the liver. *Melanoma Res*. 2004;14:67–72.
33. Mavligit GM, Charnsangavej C, Carrasco CH, et al. Regression of ocular melanoma metastatic to the liver after hepatic arterial chemoembolization with cisplatin and polyvinyl sponge. *JAMA*. 1988;260:974–976.
34. Leyvraz S, Spataro V, Bauer J, Pampallona S, Salmon R, Dorval T, Meuli R, Gillet M, Lejeune F, Zografos L. Treatment of ocular melanoma metastatic to the liver by hepatic arterial chemotherapy. *J Clin Oncol*. 1997;15:2589–2595.
35. Poon RT, Fan ST, Lo CM, Ng IO, Liu CL, Lam CM, Wong J. Improving survival results after resection of hepatocellular carcinoma: a prospective study of 377 patients over 10 years. *Ann Surg*. 2001;234:63–70.
36. Lee NW, Wong J, Ong GB. The surgical management of primary carcinoma of the liver. *World J Surg*. 1982;6:66–75.
37. Feldman ED, Wu PC, Gnant MXF, Bartlett DL, Libutti SK, Pingpank JF, Alexander HR Jr. Treatment of patients with unresectable primary hepatic malignancies using hyperthermic isolated hepatic perfusion. *J GI Surg*. 2004;8:200–207.
38. Hafström LR, Holmberg SB, Naredi PLJ, Lindnér PG, Bengtsson A, Tidebrant G, Scherstén TSO. Isolated hyperthermic liver perfusion with chemotherapy for liver malignancy. *Surg Oncol*. 1994;3:103–108.
39. Grover AC, Libutti SK, Pingpank JF, Helsabeck C, Beresnev T, Alexander HR Jr. Isolated hepatic perfusion for the treatment of patients with advanced liver metastases from pancreatic and gastrointestinal neuroendocrine neoplasms. *Surgery*. 2004;136:1176–1182.
40. Hafström L, Naredi P. Isolated hepatic perfusion with extracorporeal oxygenation using hyperthermia TNFα and melphalan: Swedish experience. *Recent Results Cancer Res*. 1998;147:120–126.
41. Lindner P, Fjalling M, Hafström L, Nielsen H, Mattson H. Isolated hepatic perfusion with extracorporeal oxygenation using hyperthermia tumour necrosis factor alpha and melphalan. *Eur J Surg Oncol*. 1999;25:179–185.
42. Pingpank JF, Libutti SK, Chang R, Wood BJ, Neeman Z, Seidel G, Alexander HR. A phase I feasibility study of hepatic arterial melphalan infusion with hepatic arterial melphalan infusion with hepatic venous hemofiltration using percutaneously placed catheters in patients with unresectable hepatic malignancies. *Am Soc Clin Oncol Proc*. 2003;22:282 (Abstract)
43. Marinelli A, Vahrmeijer AL, van de Velde CJ. Phase I/II studies of isolated hepatic perfusion with mitomycin C or melphalan in patients with colorectal cancer hepatic metastases. *Recent Results Cancer Res*. 1998;147:83–94.
44. Alexander HR Jr, Bartlett DL, Libutti SK, Fraker DL, Moser T, Rosenberg SA. Isolated hepatic perfusion with tumor necrosis factor and melphalan for unresectable cancers confined to the liver. *J Clin Oncol*. 1998;16:1479–1489.
45. Vahrmeijer AL, Van Dierendonck JH, Keizer HJ, Beijnen JH, Tollenaar RA, Pijl ME, Marinelli A, Kuppen PJ, van Bockel JH, Mulder GJ, van de Velde CJ. Increased local cytostatic drug exposure by isolated hepatic perfusion: a phase I clinical and pharmacologic evaluation of treatment with high dose melphalan in patients with colorectal cancer confined to the liver. *Br J Cancer*. 2000;82:1539–1546.

Management of Common Bile Duct Stones in the Era of Laparoscopic Surgery

CLAUDE SMADJA, NADA HELMY, and ALESSIO CARLONI
Department of Digestive Surgery, Hôpital Antoine Béclère, Université Paris

1.   INTRODUCTION

In the era of laparoscopic surgery, the best approach for common bile duct (CBD) stones remains a matter of debate. When CBD exploration was performed by laparotomy, prospective randomized trials did not show the superiority of preoperative endoscopic sphincterotomy (ES) over CBD surgery for stones.[1,2] The advent of laparoscopic surgery led to a dramatic change in the approach of CBD stones treatment. Indeed, because of an obvious lack of expertise in laparoscopic surgery, surgeons elected to detect and treat preoperatively CBD stones by ES since they considered laparoscopic CBD exploration as an unduly, complex, and demanding procedure. It is worth mentioning that this approach requires several sessions of anesthesia and cumulates the risk of ES and laparoscopic cholecystectomy. In addition, it increases the cost.[3,4] About 15 years after the introduction of laparoscopic cholecystectomy, one has to wonder whether or not this policy should be still applied. Indeed, in patients fit for surgery, laparoscopic CBD stones extraction seems to be superior to the association of ES and laparoscopic cholecystectomy.[5] The reported incidence of CBD stones found during laparoscopic cholecystectomy ranges from 3 to 10%.[6-8] It is unclear whether an asymptomatic choledocholithiasis requires treatment. Furthermore, it is well established that small stones may pass through the ampulla of Vater.[9] Moreover, it is not clear what stone size precludes transpapillary migration into the duodenum nor which criteria will predict complications of pancreatitis or cholangitis if CBD stones are not treated. Therefore, it is generally recommended to treat CBD stones whenever detected. Theoretically, CBD stones can be treated with or without cholecystectomy. Moreover, if cholecystectomy is performed this could be done before, during or after CBD stones extraction. The purpose of this chapter is to try to clarify these different points.

2.   CBD STONES EXTRACTION WITHOUT CHOLECYSTECTOMY

Treatment of CBD stones without cholecystectomy appears to be the most simple non surgical approach. But what happens when the gallbladder has been left in situ? In two randomized trials in which open CBD surgery was compared to ES, 20% of the patients managed expectantly after ES needed cholecystectomy during follow-up.[10,11] These results have been confirmed by Boerma et al.[12] These authors showed in a prospective randomized

N. A. Habib and R. Canelo (eds.), Liver and Pancreatic Diseases Management, 17–22.
© 2006 *Springer. Printed in The Netherlands.*

trial that after ES in patients fit for surgery, a wait-and-see policy concerning cholelithiasis was not valid. Indeed, with a median follow-up of 30 months, patients treated for CBD stones by ES without cholecystectomy had, in 50% of cases, biliary symptoms. Eighty percent of these patients had finally a cholecystectomy, suggesting that such a policy could not be recommended.

3.   CBD STONES DETECTION

Identifying patients with CBD stones remains a diagnostic challenge. Indeed, CBD stones detection can be realized preoperatively or intraoperatively. In addition, in the preoperative period, screening can be systematic or selective. A systematic preoperative detection of CBD stones by ERCP has been assessed by Neuhaus et al.[13] In a prospective study, they showed that 11% of the patients undergoing ERCP had CBD stones. Seventy percent of them had arguments in favor of CBD stones before ERCP on clinical and biological grounds, whereas 30% did not. According to the results of this study, there is no strong argument which allows to propose a systematic preoperative detection of CBD stones. Should this policy be selective? In a prospective study, Widdison et al.[14] assessed the place of selective preoperative ERCP. In their work, ERCP was performed in patients with either abnormal liver function tests, CBD diameter superior 3–8 mm, a past history of jaundice or an episode of acute pancreatitis. CBD stones were present in less than 50% of the patients except in the group of patients suffering from jaundice, in which the rate was 87%. Therefore, according to the results of this study, it is not recommended to adopt a policy of selective preoperative detection of CBD stones. In the same way, Montariol et al.[15] evaluated, in a prospective study, the value of a policy of selective detection of CBD stones in patients with symptomatic cholelithiasis, but without signs suggestive of the presence of CBD stones. To be included in their study, patients were selected on the basis of a predictive score of CBD stones. Patients with a score greater than 3.5, corresponding to a risk of CBD stones superior to 25%,[16] had an endoscopic ultrasonography (EUS) and an intraoperative cholangiography (IOC), while those with a score inferior to 3.5 did not, since in this population, the risk of CBD stones is estimated to be less than 5%. This study showed that when both investigations were positive, there were 5% of false positive. At the opposite, when both investigations were negative, there were no false negative. Interestingly, when the results of EUS and IOC were discordant, 86% of false negative and 100% of false positive were always due to EUS. The results of this study allowed the authors to conclude that IOC was superior to preoperative EUS for the detection of CBD stones. Finally, the best strategy is to detect CBD stones intraoperatively using IOC[17] or more recently by intraoperative ultrasonsography.[18] This approach was validated by Huguier et al.[17] in a multivariate analysis. These authors set up a formula taking into account several parameters (age of the patient, CBD diameter, size of stones, presence of a previous history of biliary colic, and cholecystitis). They showed that when the score calculated using their formula was inferior to 3.5, the probability of CBD stones was 2%. This probability was 81% when the score was superior to 5.9 and 17% when the score was comprised between 3.5 and 5.9. More recently, the use of simple predictive criteria adapted to the age of the patient has been proposed.[19] In the era of laparoscopic cholecystectomy, IOC should be performed in selected cases. When CBD stones are detected, CBD exploration should be performed and clearance obtained. In case of failure of extraction, what should be done? In other words, should the procedure be converted to laparotomy or post ES performed? In a prospective randomized trial of Rhodes et al.,[20] patients were randomly allocated to laparoscopic cholecytstectomy and CBD stones extraction or to laparoscopic cholecystectomy followed by postoperative ES. This study showed that the rate of CBD stones clearance was similar in both groups (laparoscopic CBD stones extraction: 100% vs. postoperative ES:93%). This study suggests that in case of failure of laparoscopic CBD stones extraction, postoperative ES is an acceptable option instead of conversion to open surgery.

4.   INDICATIONS OF ES

Although, ES may lead to life threatening complications such as bleeding (2%), acute pancreatitis (2%), duodenal perforation (1%), and late papillotomy stenosis (15%),[21] however, in medical practice there are still good indications of preoperative or postoperative ES. Namely when the patient had already undergone a cholecystectomy. Basically, preoperative ES should be proposed in patients with a past history of complex upper abdominal surgery: for instance a Bilroth II procedure; severe extra hepatic portal hypertension in which CBD exposure can be hazardous and the source of brisk bleeding. Finally, in the presence of acute cholecystitis. In such a situation, in some cases, inflammatory alterations of the hepatic pedicle may render impossible CBD exposure and therefore, represent a good indication of postoperative ES.

5.   SURGICAL GUIDELINES

The laparoscopic treatment of CBD stones is safe.[8,22–24] In essence, CBD stones can be removed via the cystic duct or through choledochotomy. Cystic duct extraction which is preferentially used by a large majority of surgeons[25–27] is a very simple procedure. This approach is limited by the anatomic features of the cystic duct, especially when it joins downwards the CBD in the retro-duodenal area or on its left aspect. Furthermore, it carries several disadvantages. Indeed, bile duct injury can be created while dilating the cystic duct, in order to allow the introduction of the flexible endoscope or if the CBD stone is larger than the lumen of the cystic duct. Moreover, because of the angulation of the cystic duct at the junction with the CBD, in most cases, upper biliary endoscopy appears to be technically impossible and can lead to a higher rate of retained stones, although in some studies, the retained stone rate is inferior to 1%.[25,28] The transcystic approach is indicated in case of small stones in a limited number with a large cystic duct with a modal implantation. It is worth mentioning that in the transcystic duct approach, stones smaller than 3 to 4 mm in size can often be flushed through the ampulla into the duodenum, which is facilitated by relaxation of the sphincter of Oddi using intravenous glucagon.[29] When this method fails, a Dormia basket can be passed through the cystic duct and into the CBD to extract stones. If attempts at transcystic Dormia basket extraction fail, a flexible endoscope should be inserted to remove the stones under direct vision. The flexible endoscope is passed through a midaxillary port. The flexible endoscope is placed into the CBD through the cystic duct under direct vision. The lumen of the duct is then visualized by infusing saline through the operator channel. Under visual guidance, the tip of the Dormia basket is advanced beyond the stone and opened. As the Dormia basket is pulled backwards and rotated the stone is ensnared and extracted by retrieving synchronously the flexible endoscope and the Dormia catheter. The success rate of the transcystic approach varies from 69 to 92%,[23,25,26] but concerns selected patients.

At the opposite, although choledochotomy is technically more complex, however, this approach allows thorough endoscopic exploration of the bile ducts. Choledochotomy should be done vertically, since it can be lengthened without any difficulty and is more easy to close than a horizontal opening. Complete clearance of the bile ducts under choledochoscopic guidance allows to close the CBD without any biliary drainage.[20,26,30] CBD closure should be performed using continuous or interrupted resorbable stiches. This approach allows to shorten the postoperative hospital stay. CBD stricture following choledochotomy has never been reported.[26,31,32] In practice, if transcystic approach fails or is not indicated, CBD is opened. Main indications for laparoscopic choledochotomy are stones which are multiple, large or located in the upper biliary tree above the cystic duct inplantation. The length of CBD opening is adapted to allow the introduction of the 5 mm flexible endoscope and removal of the largest stone. Stones are removed under endoscopic visualization. The routine use of operative choledochoscopy has allowed to decrease the rate of retained stone.[33,34] In the presence of an impacted stone, laser lithotripsy should be used, in order to avoid postoperative ES.[22] The success rate of CBD stones extraction is up to 97%.[25]

In case of failure of CBD stones extraction or if doubt persists for a possible retained stone, a thin drain (Escat drain) is placed into the CBD via the cystic duct in order to decompress the CBD. CBD opening is closed subsequently. A postoperative cystic tube cholangiography is performed and ES is realized if CBD stone is detected. The transcystic drain is then closed and removed more rapidly than a T tube drain.

6.   PRESENT RECOMMANDATIONS AND CONCLUSION

In patients fit for surgery, in most cases, there is no place for preoperative investigations to ascertain the presence of stones in the CBD. IOC is indicated in selected patients. Selection of patients is based on simple preoperative criteria. Finally, postoperative ES should be performed in patients with retained stone or when laparoscopic CBD stones extraction has failed. According to the results of the literature,[35] the success rate for ES (median 92%) and duct clearance (median 91%), the complication rate (median 8%) mortality rate (median 1%), recurrence stone rate (2–16%) which increases according to the length of follow up, are not superior to those obtained by the laparoscopic CBD approach. All efforts must be paid to simplify the preoperative investigations and to adopt an operative protocol using the laparoscopic approach, taking into account the size of the cystic duct, its anatomy features, the size and the number of CBD stones.

Nowadays, the strategy adopted in laparoscopic surgery for CBD stones is similar to that used during the era of open surgery, suggesting that in teams involved in laparoscopic surgery, the so-called learning curve of CBD stones extraction belongs to the past.

REFERENCES

1. Neoptolemos JP, Carr-Locke DL, Fossard DP. Prospective randomised study of preoperative endoscopic sphincterotomy *versus* Surgery alone for common bile duct stones. *Br Med J.* 1987;294:470–474.
2. Suc B, Escat J, Cherqui D et al. Surgery vs endoscopy as primary treatment in symptomatic patients with suspected common bile ducts stones. A multicenter randomized trial. *Arch Surg.* 1998;133:702–708.
3. Urbach DR, Khajanchee YS, Jobe BA, Standage BA, Hansen PD, Swanstrom LL. Cost-effective management of common bile duct stones. A decision analysis of the use of endoscopic retrograde cholangiopancreatography (ERCP), intraoperative cholangiography, and laparoscopic bile duct exploration. *Surg Endosc.* 2001;15:4–13.
4. Vecchio R, Mac Fadyen BV. Laparoscopic common bile duct exploration. *Langen Arch Surg.* 2002;387:45–54.
5. Cuschieri A, Lezoche E, Morino M et al. EAES multicenter prospective randomized trial comparing two-stage vs single-stage management of patients with gallstone disease and ductal calculi. *Surg Endosc.* 1999;13:952–957.
6. Barkuns JS, Barkun AN, Sampalis JS et al. Randomized controlled trial of laparoscopic versus mini-cholecystectomy. *Lancet.* 1992;340:1116–1119.
7. Frazee R, Roberts J, Symmonds R et al. Combined laparoscopic and endoscopic management of cholelithiasis and choledocholithiasis. *Am J Surg.* 1993;166:702–705.
8. Paganini AM, Lezoche E. Follow-up of 161 unselected consecutive patients treated laparoscopically for common bile duct stones. *Surg Endosc.* 1998;12:23–29.
9. Acosta JM, Ledesma CL. Gallstone migration as a cause of acute pancreatitis. *N Engl J Med.* 1974;290:484–487.
10. Hammarstrom LE, Holmin T, Strid Beck H, Ihse I. Long term follow-up of a prospective randomised study of endoscopic versus surgical treatment of bile duct calculi in patients with gallbladder in situ. *Br J Surg.* 1995;82:1516–1521.
11. Targarona EM, Perez Ayuso RM, Bordas JM et al. Randomised trial of endoscopic sphincterotomy with gallbladder left in situ versus open surgery for common bile duct calculi in high risk patients. *Lancet.* 1996;347:926–929.
12. Boerma D, Rauws EAJ, Keulemans YCA et al. Wait-and-see policy or laparoscopic cholecystectomy after endoscopic sphincterotomy for bile duct stones: a randomised trial. *Lancet.* 2002;360:761–765.
13. Neuhaus H, Feussner H, Ungeheur A, Hoffman W, Siewert JR, Classen M. Prospective evaluation of the use of endoscopic retrograde cholangiography prior to lapaorsocopic cholecystectomy. *Endoscopy.* 1992;24:745–749.
14. Widdison AL, Longstaff AJ, Armstrong CP. Combined laparoscopic and endoscopic treatment of gallstones and bile duct stones: a prospective study. *Br J Surg.* 1994;81:595–597.
15. Montariol T, Msika S, Charlier A et al. Diagnosis of asymptomatic common bile duct stones : preoperative endoscopic ultrasonography versus intraoperative cholangiography—a multicenter, prospective controlled study. *Surgery.* 1998;124: 6–13.
16. Montariol T, Rey C, Charlier A et al. Preoperative evalutation of the probability of common bile duct stones. *J Am Coll Surg.* 1995;180:293–296.
17. Huguier M, Bornet P, Charpak Y, Houry S, Chastang C. Selective contraindications based on multivariate analysis for operative cholangiography in biliary lithiasis. *Surg Gynecol Obstet.* 1991;172:470–473.
18. Catheline JM, Turner R, Paries J. Laparoscopic ultrasonography is a complement to cholangiography for the detection of choledocholithiasis at laparoscopic cholecystectomy. *Br J Surg.* 2002;89:1235–1239.
19. Prat F, Meduri B, Ducot B, Chiche R, Salimbeni-Bartolini R, Pelletier G. Prediction of common bile duct stones by noninvasive tests. *Ann Surg.* 1999;229:362–368.
20. Rhodes M, Sussman L, Cohen L, Lewis MP. Randomised trial of laparoscopic exploration of common bile duct versus postoperative endoscopic retrograde cholangiography for common bile duct stones. *Lancet.* 1998;351:159–161.
21. Cotton B. Endoscopic retrograde cholangiopancreatography and laparoscopic cholecystectomy. *Am J Surg.* 1993;165:474–478.
22. Stoker ME. Common bile duct exploration in the era of laparoscopic surgery. *Arch Surg.* 1995;130:265–269.
23. Millat B, Fingerhut A, Deleuze A et al. Prospective evaluation in 121 consecutive unselected patients undergoing laparoscopic treatment of choledocholithiasis. *Br J Surg.* 1995;82:1266–1269.

24. Dorman JP, Franklin ME Jr, Glass JL. Laparoscopic common bile duct exploration by choledochotomy: an effective and efficient method of treatment of choledocholithiasis. *Surg Endosc.* 1998;12:926–928.
25. Berthou JC, Drouard F, Charbonneau P, Moussalier K. Evaluation of laparoscopic management of common bile duct stones in 220 patients. *Surg Endosc.* 1988;12:16–22.
26. Martin IJ, Bailey IS, Rhodes M, O'Rourke N, Nathanson L, Fielding G. Towards T-tube free laparoscopic bile duct exploration. A methodologic evolution during 300 consecutive procedures. *Ann Surg* 1998;228:29–34.
27. Berci G, Morgenstern L. Laparoscopic management of common bile duct stones. A multi-institutional SAGES study. *Surg Endosc.* 1994;8:1168–1175.
28. Giurgiu DI, Margulies DR, Carroll BJ et al. Laparoscopic common bile duct exploration: long-term outcome. *Arch Surg.* 1999;134:839–844.
29. Petelin J. Laparoscopic approach to common bile duct pathology. *Surg Laparosc Endosc.* 1991;1:33–41.
30. Liberman MA, Phillips EH, Carroll BJ, Fallas MJ, Rosenthal R, Hiatt J. Cost-effective management of complicated choledocholithiasis: laparoscopic transcystic duct exploration or endoscopic sphincterotomy. *J Am Coll Surg.* 1996;182:488–494.
31. Keeling NJ, Menzies D, Motson RW. Laparoscopic exploration of the common bile duct: beyond the learning curve. *Surg Endosc.* 1999;13:109–112.
32. Croce E, Golia M, Azzola M et al. Laparoscopic choledochotomy with primary closure. Follow-up (5–44 months) of 31 patients. *Surg Endosc.* 1996;10:1064–1068.
33. Escat J, Gluksman DL, Maigne C, Fourtanier G, Fournier D, Vaislic C. Choledochoscopy in surgery for choledocholithiasis. Six years experience in 380 consecutive patients. *Am J Surg.* 1984;147:670–671.
34. Phillips EH, Carroll BJ, Pearlstein AR, Daykhousky L, Fallas MJ. Laparoscopic choledochoscopy and extraction of common bile duct stones. *World J Surg.* 1993;17:22–28.
35. Tranter SE, Thompson MH. Comparison of endoscopic sphincterotomy and laparoscopic exploration of the common bile duct. *Br J Surg.* 2002;89:1495–1504.

Split-Liver Transplantation

HANS JUERGEN SCHLITT, MARTIN ROSS, and AIMAN OBED
Department of Surgery, University of Regensburg Medical Center, 93057 Regensburg, Germany

1. INTRODUCTION

Donor organ shortage with the resulting restrictions in indication for liver transplantation as well as a considerable mortality on the waiting lists are major clinical problems. This has led to various approaches to increasing the number of transplantable grafts, e.g. the use of marginal donor organs, the splitting of cadaveric grafts, as well as the application of living-related partial liver transplantation. The latter two methods are based on similar techniques of liver dissection, and have, therefore, developed almost in parallel.

The technique of cutting down liver grafts dates back to the early 1980s when partial liver grafts (usually left-lateral lobes) were used for transplanting small children.[1] In these days, the rest of the liver used to be sacrificed just for obtaining a small graft suitable for a pediatric patient. With increasing expertise in liver resection techniques as well as improving results in liver transplantation this has then led to the first split-liver transplantation, performed by Rudolf Pichlmayr in Hannover in early 1988.[2] In the same year Henri Bismuth in Paris has also performed a split-liver transplantation using an independently developed similar technique. In both cases one part of the graft was used for a pediatric patient, while the other was transplanted into an adult.

Over the following years split-liver transplants were performed only sporadically, mostly in cases where two critically ill recipients required urgent transplantation.[3] Due to this selection of high-risk candidates, the overall results of split-liver transplantation were inferior to whole organ transplantation. It was not before the early to mid-1990s that several groups adopted the concept for elective cases and showed results that were almost identical to standard liver transplantation. In the mid to late 1990s many centers worldwide started programs of split-liver transplantation, in the majority of cases serving one child (left-lateral lobe) and one adult (extended right lobe).[4,5] At the same time, some centers also started to perform split-liver transplantation for two adults, preferentially using a right and a left lobe, but results with this approach have been ambivalent.[4] While, splitting the liver for one child and one adult is now considered as a standard procedure, splitting for two adults still remains experimental and is limited to highly selected cases (generally small adults in stable condition).

In terms of nomenclature it has to be considered that some authors use the term "split liver transplantation" also for partial liver transplantation from living donors; this manuscript, however, focuses selectively on split-liver transplantation from deceased donors.

N. A. Habib and R. Canelo (eds.), Liver and Pancreatic Diseases Management, 23–28.
© 2006 *Springer. Printed in The Netherlands.*

Table 1. Factors influencing the decision about splitting

Donor parameters
    age, time on ICU, sodium, ASAT, γGT, cause of death, hemodynamic stability
Intraoperative parameters
    macroscopic appearance, anatomic variants
Logistic parameters
    in-situ/ex-situ splitting, donor hospital, availability of experienced surgeon
Recipient parameters
    HU-situation/critical recipient, recipient size/weight

1.1.   Technique

Successful liver splitting and subsequent split-liver transplantation requires thorough consideration and evaluation whenever an organ donor is available. The decision about whether or not to split a donor liver—and if yes, whether to do it in-situ or ex-situ—depends on a number of variables which have different degrees of impact on decision-making.[6] These variables include formal donor-related data, the given anatomic situation, the macroscopic appearance of the liver, the weight and clinical state of the potential recipients, the availability of an experienced surgeon, and a number of logistic aspects (Table 1). An ideal liver to split (Table 2) would be from a young donor with no history of liver disease or damage, with normal liver values (particularly the γ-glutamyl-transpeptidase (γGT)), and short intensive care (ICU) time, who is hemodynamically stable before and during the donor operation. Macroscopically, the liver should have a soft consistency, be sharp-edged, and preferably have a large left-lateral lobe (unless the recipient of this part is a very small child); a separate left hepatic artery is advantageous. For optimal logistics, this donor should be explanted in the transplant center itself, thus providing optimal conditions for in-situ splitting. Unfortunately, these criteria are fulfilled only by a small minority of the currently available organ donors. Therefore, compromises are necessary in clinical practice.

A basis of all splitting procedures is the segmental anatomy of the liver with rather standardized—although somewhat variable—branching of the portal pedicles (artery, portal vein, bile duct) and hepatic veins. According to the time-point and the setting of splitting, two different techniques can be distinguished: splitting "ex-situ", i.e. on the backtable in the ice-bath after perfusion and harvesting of the whole liver, sometimes also called "ex-vivo";

Table 2. Optimal donor parameters for liver splitting

Young, healthy donor (<40(−50) years of age)
No history of liver disease/damage
Normal liver enzymes (ASAT, ALAT, γGT)
Short ICU time (≤2 days)
Hemodynamic stability
Macroscopically normal liver

and splitting "in-situ", i.e. inside the heart-beating donor prior to perfusion and harvesting of the liver (parts), sometimes also called "in-vivo". According to the line of splitting, again two different types can be distinguished: extended-right lobe (including segment I) and left-lateral lobe splitting, generally used for one child and one adult; and full right-/left-lobe splitting, mostly aimed at transplanting two adults. Both types of splitting can principally be performed "ex-situ" as well as "in-situ".

While in the early days splitting was performed ex-situ, i.e. after perfusion and harvesting of the organ and transport back to the transplant center where the surgical procedure was done on the backtable, in-situ has become more popular in the 1990s. With growing experience also with living-related liver transplantation, in-situ splitting techniques—which are almost identical to what is also done in living donors, has been strongly advocated by several groups.[5,7] Both procedure have advantages as well as disadvantages, and nowadays both techniques coexist and are applied according to the individual situation. Advantages of the ex-situ-procedure are mostly of logistical nature. A standard team can perform the organ retrieval at any hospital without any delay, while the (more elaborate) splitting procedure is done "at home" under optimal conditions. Thus, it can even be used in the case of a non-heart-beating donor.[8] This is, however, associated with a relevant increase in cold ischemic time, and also with some warming up of the graft during backtable perparation. A higher risk of graft dysfunction after transplantation may be induced by these circumstances, but there are no solid data on that.[9] Another disadvantage of ex-situ splitting is the inability to evalute the perfusion and venous drainage of certain parts of the liver, e.g. perfusion of segment IV in case of extended-right/left-lateral splitting or the venous drainage of segment V in full right/left splitting. Moreover, the completeness of hemostasis on the resection surface is not guaranteed when using this technique. On the other hand, in-situ splitting has the advantage to be associated with a short ischemic time and with a completely dry resection surface, and it allows a clear judgment of the perfusion situation (with the potential to decide whether or not to reconstruct certain vessels).[10] The logistics of in-situ splitting are, however, much more difficult. Particularly, with a donor not being hospitalized in the transplant center, but in a peripheral hospital, the organization can be difficult. A highly experienced surgical team has to be available; the surgical conditions may not be optimal with limited equipment provided there; and it requires additional surgical time in a situation where those peripheral hospitals may be at the limits of their willingness to cooperate because the donor operation interferes with their own surgical activities anyway. For the in-situ splitting, two types of perfusion are possible: either the left lateral segment is taken out perliminarily and perfused ex-situ (as for living-related liver transplantation), or the whole liver is perfused in-situ after dissection of the parenchyma and the vessels are divided afterwards in an "a-la carte" fashion.

So far, most splitting procedure have been done to serve one child and one adult by splitting the liver basically along the falciform ligament, creating a left-lateral lobe of around 250–300 g and an extended right lobe graft (including segment I) of about 1,300 g in case of a "normal" liver. The division of the hilar structures may vary slightly from center to center, but mostly, the left-lateral lobe is harvested with the left hepatic artery, the left portal vein branch (if possible, distal to a major segement I-branch) as well as the left-lateral bile duct (or ducts) distal to the segment IV duct; maintainance of the left hepatic veins leaves optimal venous drainage of the graft in essentially all cases so that small venous branches draining to the middle hepatic vein can be ligated. In terms of the artery, some centers prefer keeping the celiac axis with the left lateral graft and have only the right artery with the right extended graft in order to provide optimal conditions for arterial reconstruction for the pediatric part. Currently, extended-right/left-lateral splitting has become a routine procedure in many centers and should be taken into consideration whenever possible. The techniques for this type of splitting are more or less standardized so that many centers even rely on (experienced) foreign teams to perform the splitting and to accept such a partial graft after shipping.

In contrast, full right/left splitting is still a more experimental procedure and is suitable only for rather small adults. The techniques still vary considerably between the few involved centers. Most surgeons advocate leaving the middle hepatic vein with the (usually smaller and thereby more critical) left lobe[11] or using even a "split cava" technique to obtain optimal venous drainage for both parts.[12] For this type of splitting, the in-situ technique seems to be clearly favorable in order to avoid additional damage to the grafts by extended cold ischemic time. In principle, the techniques are very similar to the procedure performed for right lobe living donation.

2.   RESULTS

For pediatric recipients, split-liver transplantation presents an alternative to full-size pedatric liver transplantation and with living-donor transplantation. While full-size transplantation in pediatric patients is rarely possible due to the scarcity of size-matched donor organs available, split-liver and living-donor transplantation have to be evalutated against each other because both can be discussed in almost all patients. In terms of logisti-cal and medical issues, living-donor transplantation might be preferred because it allows a scheduled transplantation at an optimal timing with a (regularly) very good organ. Although it has proved to be a generally very safe technique, it is associated with some morbidity and even some mortality (although with a risk of <0.1% in experienced centers) in the living donors. In fact, a wide-spread use of split-liver transplantation using carefully se-lected optimal donor organs (see above), could provide enough left-lateral grafts in order to transplant all pediatric patients in need within few weeks—a time frame that is suffi-cient in most cases.[13] This, of course, leads to the discussion about short-term as well as long-term results of the various techniques in pediatric patients. Although some centers have suggested slightly improved results with living-donor transplantation, most programs show that with adequate donor selection, improved logistics, and meticulous technique, both procedures lead to similarly good results in terms of patient and graft survival,[7,10,14,15] although early graft function may be slightly worse after split-liver transplantation.[16] Over-all, however, there does not seem to be a major advantage of living donation so that—at least in Europe and the United States, where organs from deceased donors are quite readily available, split-liver transplantation should be the first choice for pediatric patients. Since the extended-right lobe still remains for transplantation of an adult patient, a policy of aggressive splitting would strongly help pediatric patients while not giving a disadvan-tage to adult patients on the waiting lists; such a policy should, therefore, be strongly encouraged.

For adult recipients of extended right lobe grafts (i.e. the "left-over" from a pediatric graft) it has been shown—particularly in the early phase – that there is an increased risk for vascular as well as biliary complications.[4,10,17] Specifically, the perfusion of segment IV may be suboptimal in some patients and can then be associated with partial necrosis and a bile leak in that area. Although in most cases such problems can be managed interventionally, i.e. without operation, they are associated with an increased morbidity. However, more recent data, including rather large series from experienced centers, have shown that with adequate patient selection and careful technique, the complication rates can be very low and results comparable with that of whole organ transplantation.[13] Overall, there is probably a higher risk of morbidity and mortality for the patients after transplantation with a marginal whole organ as compared to an optimal split liver graft—although no randomized studies exist (and will probably ever exist) on that issue.

The data on the results of full right/left lobe liver splitting for two adults are more heterogeneous.[11,18,19] Of particular concern remains the rather low volume of the graft which puts the recipient at a considerable risk of a small-for-size syndrome with subsequent liver failure. While quite inferior results were initially reported by some centers evaluating such techniques, it was recently demonstrated that with very careful selection of donors and recipients, and with very careful technique, good results can be achieved with this approach—at least in highly selected centers.

Overall, it has to be kept in mind that the use of split livers (or other type of "less than optimal" grafts) is always associated with a certain increase in risk for the patient. Therefore, the use of split livers in adult patients should be usually restricted to rather stable patients. A critically ill patient needs as much liver mass and transplant safety as possible, because early dysfunction or even slight complications may put him at a serious risk, while a stable patient will be able to cope with that. The inferior results obtained in adults in the early phase of liver splitting were to large parts due to the fact that it was frequently applied in critical situations, e.g. when urgent transplantion of two critically ill patients was required when only one graft was available. If these situations are avoided, split-liver transplantation can give excellent results for adults as well.

Once the liver function has started sufficiently, growth and regeneration of the partial grafts in the recipients appear to be very rapid. Systematic studies by CT scans after transplantation have shown that after 3 months, the grafts have generally grown to more than 100% of the patients' "ideal liver volume" both after living donation as well as after split-liver transplantation, no matter whether right or left grafts were used.[20] Thus, transplanting a suboptimal mass of liver does not appear to be associated with inferior long-term results.

3. CONCLUSION

Over the last 15 years, split-liver transplantation has become a technique applied by many transplant centers around the world. So far, it is predominantly used for transplanting one child and one adult with the two parts of one donor liver. Although slightly different techniques are used by different centers, the extended right/left-lateral splitting is rather standardized and is performed either ex-situ or in-situ. While the in-situ approach appears to be superior in medical terms, the ex-situ technique has logistical advantages so that the decision must be made in dependence of each individual setting. Splitting of a donor liver for two adults is still an experimental procedure and limited to selected centers.

In summary, split-liver transplantation is a technically demanding procedure, but well performed, it can lead to good results. In conjunction with living donor liver transplantation as well as the use of marginal donor organs from deceased donors, it offers the chance to extend the number of available donor organs and, thereby, to reduce the mortality on the waiting lists for liver transplantation.

REFERENCES

1. Broelsch CE, Emond JC, Thistlethwaite JR, et al. Liver transplantation with reduced-size donor organs. *Transplantation*. 1988;45:519–524.
2. Pichlmayr R, Ringe B, Gubernatis G, et al. Transplantation of a donor liver to 2 recipients (splitting transplantation)—a new method in the further development of segmental liver transplantation. *Langenbecks Arch Chir.* 1988;373:127–130.
3. Broelsch CE, Emond JC, Whitington PF, et al. Application of reduced-size liver transplants as split grafts, auxiliary grafts, and living related segmental transplants. *Ann. Surg.* 1990;212:368–375.
4. Azoulay D, Astarcioglu I, Bismuth H, et al. Split-liver transplantation. The Paul Brousse policy. *Ann. Surg.* 1996;224:737–746.
5. Rogiers X, Malago M, Gawad K, et al. In situ splitting of cadaveric livers. The ultimate expansion of a limited donor pool. *Ann. Surg.*1996;224:331–339.
6. Schlitt HJ. Which liver is splitable? In: Rogiers X, et al. eds. Split-Liver Transplantation—Theoretical and Practical Aspects. Darmstadt, Germany: Steinkopff Verlag; 2002:63–66.
7. Yersiz H, Renz JF, Farmer DG, Hisatake GM, McDiarmid SV, Busuttil RW. One hundred in situ split-liver transplantations: a single-center experience. *Ann. Surg.* 2003;238:496–505.
8. Muiesan P, Girlanda R, Baker A, Rela M, Heaton N. Successful segmental auxiliary liver transplantation from a non-heart-beating donor: implications for split-liver transplantation. *Transplantation*. 2003;75:1443–1445.
9. Noujaim HM, Gunson B, Mayer DA, et al. Worth continuing doing ex situ liver graft splitting? A single-center analysis. *Am. J. Transplant*. 2003;3:318–323.
10. Reyes J, Gerber D, Mazariegos GV, et al. Split-liver transplantation: a comparison of ex vivo and in situ techniques. *J. Pediatr. Surg.* 2000;35:283–289.
11. Azoulay D, Castaing D, Adam R, et al. Split-liver transplantation for two adult recipients: feasibility and long-term outcomes. *Ann. Surg.* 2001;233:565–574.
12. Gundlach M, Broering D, Topp S, Sterneck M, Rogiers X. Split-cava technique: liver splitting for two adult recipients. *Liver Transpl.* 2000;6:703–706.
13. Gridelli B, Spada M, Petz W, et al. Split-liver transplantation eliminates the need for living-donor transplantation in children with end-stage cholestatic liver disease. *Transplantation*. 2003;75:1197–1203.
14. Renz JF, Emond JC, Yersiz H, Ascher NL, Busuttil RW. Split-liver transplantation in the United States: outcomes of a national survey. *Ann. Surg.* 2004;239:172–181.
15. Deshpande RR, Bowles MJ, Vilca-Melendez H, et al. Results of split liver transplantation in children. *Ann. Surg.* 2002;236:248–253.
16. Farmer DG, Yersiz H, Ghobrial RM, et al. Early graft function after pediatric liver transplantation: comparison between in situ split livers grafts and living-related liver grafts. *Transplantation*. 2001;72:1795–1802.
17. Broering DC, Topp S, Schaefer U, et al. Split liver transplantation and risk to the adult recipient: analysis using matched pairs. *J. Am. Coll. Surg.* 2002;195:648–657.
18. Sommacale D, Farges O, Ettorre GM, et al. In situ split liver transplantation for two adult recipients. *Transplantation*. 2000;69:707–708.
19. Humar A, Ramcharan T, Sielaff TD, et al. Split liver transplantation for two adult recipients: an itial experience. *Am. J. Transplant*. 2001;1:366–372.
20. Human A, Kosari K, Sielaff TD, et al. Liver regeneration after adult living donor and deceased donor split-liver transplantation. *Liver Transpl.* 2004;10:374–378.

Surgery and Chemotherapy Combined for Colorectal Liver Metastases

BERNARD NORDLINGER

Hospital Ambroise Paré, Boulogne, University of Paris, France

1. INTRODUCTION

With time, liver metastases from colorectal cancer have become the most frequent indication for partial liver resections. Many large series of liver resection for metastatic colon cancer have been published. With progress in surgical technique and improved surgical skill, operative mortality has come down well below 5%.

The benefit of surgical resection of liver metastases has not been demonstrated by any randomized trial due to the observation that 25–30% of patients could survive 5 years after complete resection of metastasis, whereas there were very few survivors at 3 years in unresected patients in historical series.

With time, surgeons have become more aggressive. In the beginning, only solitary small unilobar metastases were resected. Progressively, indications have been extended to larger tumors, to multiple unilobar metastases and later to multiple bilobar metastases and to associated hepatic and extra hepatic deposits as long as they could be entirely removed.

Unfortunately, recurrences are still observed in two-thirds of patients after resection of liver metastases. Various attempts are being made to reduce this risk. One way would be to improve selection of patients in whom surgery is considered. The trend is rather to be more aggressive and to increase the indication for surgical resection of liver metastases rather than the opposite. Long survivals are now observed after resection of large or multiple liver metastases, in patients to whom surgery would have been refused some years ago.

Probably the most promising way to improve outcome after surgical resection of liver metastases of colorectal origin and cure more patients is to combine surgery with chemotherapy.[1]

Conclusions of a study conducted by Kemeny et al. were that hepatic artery infusion (HAI) with FUDR combined with IV continuous 5FU reduced the risk of recurrence when compared to surgery alone, but resulted in no benefit in overall survival. Two other recently published studies have evaluated the potential benefit of HAI as adjuvant treatment after resection of colorectal liver metastases. Lorenz et al. used HAI with 5FU and folinic acid without systemic treatment and showed no benefit over surgery alone. Moreover, significant toxicity was observed in patients receiving chemotherapy. The study from the Memorial Sloan Kettering Cancer Center compared HAI + systemic 5FU and folinic acid to systemic 5FU and folinic acid only and concluded that combined treatment resulted in a decrease in the hepatic recurrence rate and an improved overall survival only at 2 years.[3]

N. A. Habib and R. Canelo (eds.), Liver and Pancreatic Diseases Management, 29–30.
© 2006 *Springer. Printed in The Netherlands.*

In these studies the majority of patients could not receive the total dose, demonstrating that feasibility of HAI is not perfect.

Thus HAI alone is not sufficient as adjuvant treatment for liver metastases. HAI associated with systemic chemotherapy can reduce the risk of recurrences after surgery for liver metastases, but this potential benefit is counterbalanced by a significant rate of side effects. A widespread use of HAI as adjuvant treatment after hepatectomy is also limited by availability of FUDR and the high cost of infusion pumps. Two studies of adjuvant chemotherapy with 5FU-LV for 6 months have been reported at ASCO 2002. No statistically significant benefit was observed in the chemotherapy arm over the surgery only arm. Chemotherapy has evolved.

Whether the best timing for the administration of chemotherapy is before or after surgery or both, we do not know. Whether the best regimen should contain FUDR, 5FU, oxaliplatin, irinotecan, or other new drugs we do not know. Whether it should be administrated through the systemic or the intraarterial route we do not know either. But it is likely that the association of surgery and chemotherapy will be validated as the best treatment of resectable liver metastases in the future. In the meanwhile, surgical resection without administration of chemotherapy should remain the treatment of choice for most patients, provided resection is complete. It is thus urgent that surgeons and medical oncologists participate in large prospective trials evaluating new regimens and new treatment modalities feasible in most institutions. Due to the difficulty in organizing such trials, it is likely that only multicenter trials with possibly international cooperation will help solve the question. An international intergroup study organized by the European Organization for Research and Treatment of Cancer compares surgery with or without neoadjuvant and adjuvant oxaliplatin, 5FU, and folinic acid in patients with resectable liver metastases and has a good accrual. Studies evaluating irinotecan based regimens as adjuvant treatment after resection of liver metastases are in preparation.

Metastases considered to be resectable are not the only ones which can benefit from the cooperation between surgeons and medical oncologists. The clear distinction between resectable and unresectable metastases may very soon become obsolete. Shrinkage of tumors after administration of chemotherapy may permit resection of some metastases initially considered unresectable (2). Ongoing studies explore this field. One combines 5FU and Oxaliplatin, and another 5FU-irinotecan and Oxaliplatin to determine if some metastases considered unresectable can be resected after administration of chemotherapy.

REFERENCES

1. Kemeny N, Huang Y, Cohen AM, et al. Hepatic arterial infusion of esectable metastatic colorectal carcinoma to the liver: surgical resection of hepatic metastases in combination with continuous infusion of chemotherapy: an intergroup study. *J Clin Oncol.* 2002;20:1499–1505.
2. Lorenz M, Muller HH, Schramm H, et al. Randomized trial of surgery versus surgery followed by adjuvant hepatic arterial infusion with 5-FU and folinic acid for liver metastases of colorectal cancer. *Ann Surg.* 1998;228:756–762.
3. Kemeny N, Huang Y, Cohen AM, et al. Hepatic arterial infusion of chemotherapy after resection of hepatic metastases from colorectal cancer. *N Engl J Med.* 1999;341:2039–2048.

Radio Frequency Assisted Liver Resection: The Habib's Technique

LONG R. JIAO, GUISSEPE NAVARRA, JEAN-CHRISTOPHER
WEBER, ROMAN HAVLIC, JOANNA P. NICHOLLS,
and NAGY A. HABIB
*Department of Surgical Oncology and Technology, Imperial College School of Medicine,
London W12 0NN, UK*

1.   INTRODUCTION

Liver resection presently demands high surgical skills that take many years to acquire. Minimization of perioperative blood loss has been a major concern as this significantly influences postoperative morbidity and mortality, and long term survival.[1] Radio frequency ablation (RFA) has increasingly been used in liver surgery treating unresectable tumors.[2-4] The principle of this technique is to generate ionic agitation and frictional heating thus to lead to coagulative necrosis.[5] The clinical application of this technique in liver surgery, so far, has been the direct insertion of a radio frequency (RF) probe into tumors to achieve necrosis within the cancer cells in either primary or secondary liver cancer.[2,6] To maximize the potential benefit of this technique, a new liver resection technique assisted by the application of RF has been developed in our unit to achieve a combination of reduction of blood loss and turmoricidal effect at the resection.

2.   SURGICAL TECHNIQUE

For RF assisted liver resection, a RF a 500 kHz-RF Generator (model RFG-3D—Radionics Europe, N.V., Wettdren, Belgium) is used. A detailed description of this technique with schematic diagrams and illustrations is here given.

2.1.   Marking the Edge of Tumor

Using argon diathermy, the first line is drawn on the liver capsule along the edge of tumor to mark the periphery (Fig. 1). This is assisted by a combination of bimanual palpation and intraoperative ultrasound (IOUS). It is necessary to perform this before RFA as it becomes difficult to identify the tumor edges on palpation once the liver parenchyma hardens following RFA. In addition, an increased echogenicity from RFA will obliterate the sensitivity of IOUS.

N. A. Habib and R. Canelo (eds.), Liver and Pancreatic Diseases Management, 31–37.
© 2006 *Springer. Printed in The Netherlands.*

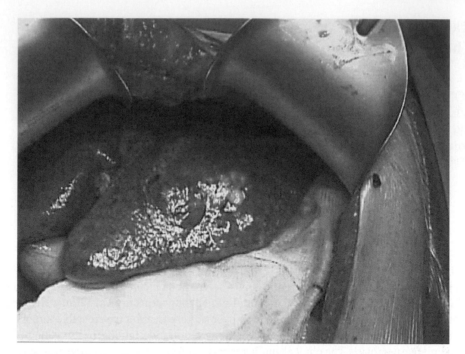

Figure 1. The first line was drawn on the liver capsule to mark the edge of the tumor.

2.2.   Marking the Site of RF Probe Insertion

A second line is created with argon diathermy 2 cm away from the first (Fig. 2). This marks the site for insertion of RF probes.

2.3.   Application of RF

A RF probe, the "cooled-tip" RF probe in our unit, is then inserted along the second line to generate coagulative necrosis (Fig. 3). This probe contains a 3 cm exposed electrode, a thermocouple on the tip to monitor temperature and impedance, and two coaxial cannulae through which chilled saline is circulated during RF energy application to prevent tissue boiling and cavitation immediately adjacent to the needle.

The number of probe applications that are required to obtain a "zone of necrosis" is related to the depth of the liver parenchyma to be resected. Each application of RF energy takes about 60 s and creates a "zone of necrosis" in a core of tissue measuring 1 cm radius by 3 cm in depth. Thus, to obtain a 12 cm core of tissue in depth four applications will be needed in vertical successions.

Application of the RF energy should begin with the area deepest and farthest from the upper surface of the liver. The position of each probe is checked with IOUS. The standard technique in our unit is to insert the tip of probe into the liver capsule of the inferior surface of the liver then to feel it with the middle finger of the left hand whilst holding the probe

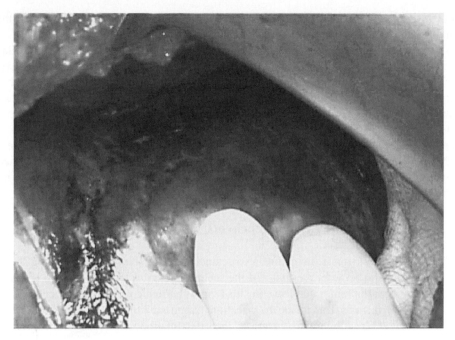

Figure 2. A second line was created 2 cm away from the first to mark the insertion site for radio frequency.

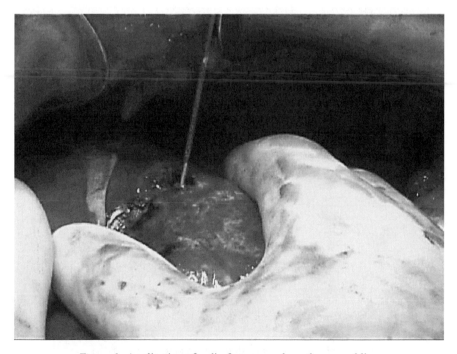

Figure 3. Application of radio frequency along the second line.

with the right hand. The areas of coagulative necrosis can be monitored using IOUS that visualizes changes in tissue impedance and formation of microbubbles in the tissue.

Once the deepest tissue is coagulated, the probe is withdrawn by 3 cm to coagulate the next cylinder of tissue and so on until the upper surface of the liver is reached. The probe is then removed and inserted into the next site which is usually 1–2 cm away from the previous application to allow complete coagulation of a band of parenchyma extending along the second line. The point of entry of each probe should be kept close to each other to achieve some overlap in order to ensure that the coagulation has been complete. Just prior to each probe removal the saline infusion is stopped to increase the temperature close to the electrode. This results in coagulation of the needle tract during withdrawal and reduces the possibility of bleeding from the probe tract and liver capsule. Pringle's maneuver is not applied with this technique.

2.4.   Division of the Liver Parenchyma

The liver parenchyma is divided using a scalpel (Fig. 4). The plane of division should be situated midway between the first and the second line so as to leave a 1 cm resection margin away from the tumor and leave in situ 1 cm of burned coagulated surface (Fig. 5).

Coagulative necrosis from inside the resection margin can be applied in order to stop any potential point of bleeding and to "increase" the safety margin particularly if the resection is to remove cancerous tissue. A drain is placed at the site of resection.

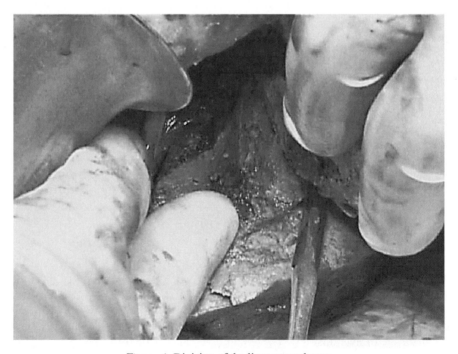

Figure 4. Division of the liver parenchyma.

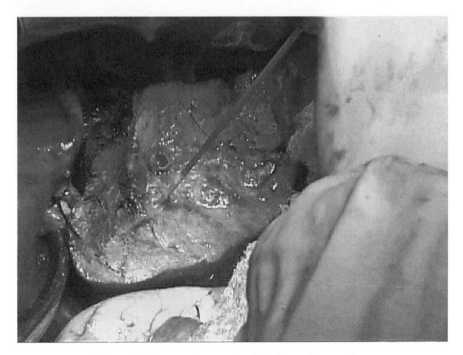

Figure 5. The resection margin of the liver after resection.

3. PATIENT AND RESULT

A 69-year-old gentleman with colorectal liver metastases underwent a segment II/III liver resection following preoperative staging with spiral computed tomography (CT) scan (Fig. 6). Under general anesthesia a modified right subcostal incision was made to expose the liver. After a formal laparotomy, which revealed no evidence of extrahepatic disease, the liver was mobilized and IOUS performed to detect any other lesions in the liver. The segmental resection was then carried out according to the steps described above. The resection time was 45 min. The total blood loss was 30 ml during the division of the liver parenchyma. There was no morbidity, and postoperatively the patient made an excellent recovery and was discharged on the day 5.

4. COMMENTS

A novel technique of liver resection assisted by RF is described here to achieve bloodless liver resection and tumoricidal effect along the resection margins without the use of sutures, surgical knots, clips, or glue. This technique allowed the segmental resection of liver metastases performed with a near zero blood loss. Technically, it is easy to learn for a surgeon with a good knowledge of liver anatomy. The length of the anesthetic time, the operating time, and the amount of blood loss can all be reduced such that it potentially minimizes the risks

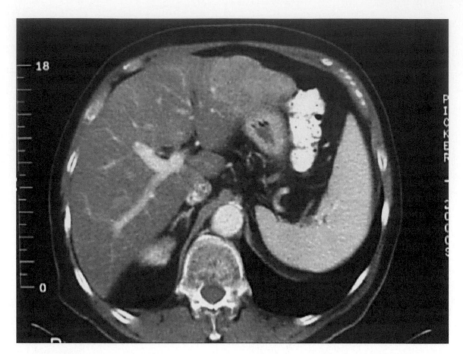

Figure 6. The preoperative CT showing liver metastases in the segment II/III.

related to liver resection, eliminates the need for intensive care unit facilities, and hence results in less postoperative mortality and morbidity. As it is a simple technique to teach it may encourage surgeons to perform more liver resections and popularize liver surgery as a "safer" therapeutic modality in the management of liver tumors. This technique will be a considerable step in making laparoscopic liver resection safer and more feasible for many liver surgeons.

The concept of using RFA in liver tumors is not new with many publications in the past few years.[2,6,7] However, the innovative step of this technique is the use of RFA in normal liver parenchyma rather than tumor mass. To achieve the effect of coagulation in normal liver parenchyma is much faster than that in tumor tissue. Typically to achieve coagulative necrosis in tumor tissue takes about 20 min for one probe application, but only 40 s to coagulate the same amount of normal liver tissue. However, there are two obvious limitations to the technique. Firstly, RF energy should be applied carefully near the hilum or the vena cava because of its damaging effect on these structures. Secondly, some "healthy" parenchymal tissue is sacrificed which is usually spared when compared with other resectional techniques. However, the regenerative capacity of residual normal tissue should mean that this disadvantage is minor.

The present method seems to offer potential additional advantages over the conventional liver resection techniques but clearly it needs to be attempted on a larger scale to compare this with other resection techniques. We venture to suggest it should be called the Habib's technique.

REFERENCES

1. Bismuth H. Major hepatic resection under total vascular exclusion. *Ann Surg*. 1989;210:13–19.
2. Jiao LR, Hansen PD, Havlic R, Mitry RR, Pignatelli M, Habib NA. Clinical short-term results of radiofrequency ablation in primary and secondary liver tumours. *Am J Surg*. 1999;177:303–306.
3. Cuschieri A, Bracken J, Boni L. Initial experience with laparoscopic ultrasound-guided radiofrequency thermal ablation of hepatic tumours. *Endoscopy*. 1999;31:318–321.
4. Curley SA, Izzo F, Delrio P, Ellis LM, Granchi J, Vallone P, Fiore F, Pignata S, Daniele B, Cremona F. Radiofrequency ablation of unresectable primary and metastatic hepatic malignancies: results in 123 patients. *Ann Surg*. 1999;230:1–8.
5. Goldberg SN, Gazelle GS, Dawson SL, Rittman WJ, Mueller PR, Rosenthal DI. Tissue ablation with radiofrequency: effect of probe size, gauge, duration and temperature on lesion volume. *Acad Radiol*. 1995;2:399–404.
6. Curley SA. Radiofrequency ablation of malignant liver tumors. *Ann Surg Oncol*. 2003;10:338–347.
7. Livraghi T, Goldberg SN, Lazzaroni S, Meloni F, Ierance T, Solbiati L, Gazelle GS. Hepatocellular carcinoma: radio-frequency ablation of medium and large lesions. *Radiology*. 2000;214:761–768.

Radio Frequency-Assisted Liver Resection: Experience of Italian Hepatic Surgery Unit

RICCARDO PELLICI, ANDREA PERCIVALE,
MICHELE PITTALUGA, MASSIMO PASQUALINI,
ALBERTO PROFETI, and ALESSANDRO PAROLDI
Department of Surgery, Santa Corona Hospital, Pietra Ligure, Savona, Italy

1.   INTRODUCTION

Radio frequency (RF) thermal ablation has increasingly been utilized for unresectable hepatic tumors. This new procedure, described by Habib and coworkers,[1,2] employs the heat produced by an RF needle electrode to obtain a previous coagulation of the tissue before cutting it and to perform a liver resection with reduced blood loss. The technical aspects, indications, and complications of the procedure are described in this chapter.

2.   MATERIAL AND METHODS

From June 2002 to July 2003, 17 patients underwent RF-assisted liver resection. There were eight women and nine male patients; mean age was 62 years (range 26–76 years). Seven patients were affected by hepatocellular carcinoma; the other nine had colorectal liver metastases and one gastric metastases. All patients received physical examination, then a preoperative computerized tomography (CT) scans of the abdomen and chest and the tumor markers title (CEA, alfa feto protein and CA 19-9) were obtained. A total of 29 tumors (range 1–3) were treated, mean dimension was 24.5 mm (range 8–60 mm). Patients received 3 left bisegmentectomies, 5 segmentectomies, and 14 wedge resections (Table 1). Four patients underwent associated intraoperative RF ablation of one liver nodule, which could not be resected. In two cases we performed a right hepatectomy and a right colectomy, respectively. Operative technique (NAH technique) is that described by the authors who first developed it. Once planned the type of hepatectomy by visual and manual exploration and liver ultrasonography (USG), the line of resection is marked by diathermy on the liver surface. The next step is the application of RF energy by a probe with 3 cm exposed end (total length 20 cm), cooled with saline solution at 0°C (Cool Tip RF, Radionics®, Burlington, MA, U.S.A.). A 480 kHz RF generator (CC1 Cosman Coagulator System, Radionics®, Burlington, MA, U.S.A.) was used; during the procedure tissue impedance, generator power output and electrode tip temperature was controlled. The needle was placed in the parenchyma under USG guidance. To obtain a zone of tissue necrosis with a 1 cm in radius and 3 cm of depth RF should last 60–90 s, confirmed by impedence value. The original procedure starts from the deepest point of the tissue of the line of resections to the most

39

N. A. Habib and R. Canelo (eds.), Liver and Pancreatic Diseases Management, 39–41.
© 2006 *Springer. Printed in The Netherlands.*

Table 1. Overview of resection vs. blood loss/ml

Patient	Segments resected	Blood loss (ml)
1	II III[a]	40
2	I II III, WR II/IV	70
3	VII, WR II, WR VIII	5
4	WR II/IV[a]	10
5	VI[a]	40
6	WR IV/VIII	5
7	WR V	150
8	WR VI	50
9	WR VIII	60
10	VII[a]	150
11	II-III-IV[a]	100
12	II[a]	10
13	WR IV (+right hepatectomy)	70
14	WR IV[a]	10
15	WR VI + WR VII	80
16	WR IV	40
17	WR VIII	20

[a] HCC.

superficial, and the number of RF sessions depends on the thickness of the parenchyma to be coagulated. We performed the procedure by needle application starting from the top face to the deepest point of the lesion to treat. After having obtained the complete coagulation of the tissue the probe is placed 2 cm away from the point of the previous application and a new one is performed: the next step is the liver resection using a common scalpel. If there is an incomplete coagulation, further RF applications can be done in specific points during the time of parenchyma resection. A prophylactic transcystic drainage (Pedinielli, PORGES S.A., Le Plessis Robinson, France) was left for 15 days in a case of V segmentectomy, because RF sessions were performed close to the main right biliary duct. An infra-hepatic drainage was always left in place.

3.   RESULTS

There were no operative deaths. Mean operative time was 220 min (range 110–420 min). Blood loss was 53 ml (range 5–150 ml), no further device (stitches, clips, tissue glue, argon beam coagulator) but RF energy was required to get adequate hemostasis. No patient received blood transfusion and Pringle maneuver was never required. One patient had an important intraoperative bleeding (total blood loss 150 ml) from an incompletely coagulated blood vessel, which was managed with manual compression and further RF sessions. Mean preoperative hemoglobin rate was 12.5 g/dl (range 9–15.9 g/dl), postoperative rate was 11.3 g/dl (range 8.5–13.4 g/dl). All patients presented a postoperative raising of the level of transaminase and bilirubin, which normalized within 10 days. Severe complications occurred in three patients (17%). Two patients developed an abscess in the site of resection after 24 and 30 days, respectively: this condition required percutaneous USG guided drainage. Another one patient developed an abscess during postoperative time; this patient underwent right emicolectomy synchronous to liver resection. These patients needed percutaneous USG guided drainage and antibiotic therapy with complete resolution. A 72-year-old patient previously affected by cardiac failure had a postoperative worsening of the disease, which was treated with drug therapy and a short stay in intensive care unit. Fever occurred in seven patients treated with short course of antipyretic drugs. Mean postoperative hospital stay was 9.4 days (range 5–20 days).

4.   DISCUSSION

RF-assisted liver resection has been developed to minimize blood losses. Hemostasis is obtained only by RF thermal energy, no further devices (stitches, knots, clips, glue etc.) are needed. In any case Pringle maneuver is not required; this can avoid liver ischemia. The line of resection treated by RF presents a coat of about 1 cm of coagulated tissue that is a further warranty for a complete resection of the neoplastic disease with negative gross margins. In order to avoid major complication as in our case (three liver abscess) it is important to reduce carefully the time of single needle application and the tissue necrosis along the resection line.

Concerning synchronous metastasis probably it is better to perform the hepatic resection in a second time to avoid easier contamination.

The main advantages of this technique remain the near-zero blood loss without inflow vascular occlusion and postoperative blood transfusion and no need to excessive hepatic mobilization. RF-assisted liver resection can be applied to both segmental and major resection: in our experience segmental resection remains the best indication particularly in cirrhotic liver while major resection still remains a challenging procedure. Further technological improvement of RF probe and generator will help us to simplify the parenchyma resection and hemostasis even though only a good knowledge of liver anatomy and function allow feasible and safe resection.[3]

REFERENCES

1. Weber JC, Navarra G, Jiao LR, Nicholls J, Jensen S, Habib NA. New technique for liver resection using heat coagulative necrosis. *Ann Surg.* 2002;236:560–563.
2. Navarra G, Spalding D, Zacharoulis D, Nicholls JP, Kirby S, Costa I, Habib NA. Bloodless hepatectomy technique. *HPB Surg.* 2002;4:95–97.
3. Regimbeau JM, Kianmanesh R, Farges O, Dondero F, Sauvanet A, Belghiti J. Extend of liver resection influences the outcome in patients with cirrhosis and small hepatocellular carcinoma. *Surgery.* 2002;13(3):311–317.

Hepatic Surgery for Metastatic Gastrointestinal Neuroendocrine Tumors

FLORENCIA G. QUE, JUAN M. SARMIENTO,
and DAVID M. NAGORNEY

*Division of Gastroenterology and General Surgery, Mayo Medical School, Mayo Clinic and
Mayo Foundation, Rochester, MN 55905, USA*

1.   INTRODUCTION

Gastrointestinal neuroendocrine cancers are of significant interest to clinicians and basic scientists. Although there have been marked improvements in the accuracy of diagnosis with improved radioimmune and hormonal assays and in the diagnosis of earlier disease by computed tomography (CT) and magnetic resonance imaging (MRI), many patients still present with hepatic metastases. In contrast to most metastatic gastrointestinal cancers, which have rapid clinical progression with a general decrease in performance status or symptoms related to visceral obstruction and pain, the progression of gastrointestinal neuroendocrine cancers is often slow and associated with clinical endocrinopathies from overproduction of gut hormones. This small subgroup of patients with metastatic neuroendocrine malignancies to the liver has become the focus of intensive multimodality therapy.

The aim of this review is to evaluate the role of cytoreductive hepatic surgery in the management of metastatic gastrointestinal malignancies. Over the last two decades, surgical techniques in both pancreatic and hepatic surgery have become reliably safe enough to broadly advocate the aggressive surgical resection of both the primary and metastatic disease whether concomitantly or sequentially. Although clinical reports on cytoreductive surgery for these tumors are sparse, our own experience supports aggressive surgical resection in selected patients with functioning metastatic neuroendocrine malignancies. Although chemotherapy has been employed, low response rates are frequent because of the decreased kinetic activity of these tumors and the high degree of tumor differentiation.

2.   RATIONALE FOR CYTOREDUCTIVE HEPATIC SURGERY

Cytoreductive surgery, defined broadly, refers to removal or in situ destruction of any tumor to reduce clinical symptoms. Clinically, however, cytoreductive hepatic surgery refers to incomplete resection of intrahepatic tumor to reduce clinical symptoms and to enhance response to additional nonsurgical therapy.[1] Cytoreductive surgery is the major component of multimodality therapy and is generally applied to incomplete gross resections. However, complete resection of all gross tumor should always be the primary aim of hepatic resection. Because the primary aim of cytoreductive hepatic surgery is to improve the quality of life, the

N. A. Habib and R. Canelo (eds.), Liver and Pancreatic Diseases Management, 43–56.
© 2006 *Springer. Printed in The Netherlands.*

risk:benefit ratio of resection must strongly favor cytoreduction. In this instance, increased survival is a secondary goal.

Cytoreductive surgery is primarily employed in tumors with few biologic characteristics that enhance the probability of a response to adjuvant therapy. Such tumor characteristics include the relatively long tumor doubling time, hepatic, and regional lymphatics as a predominant site of metastatic disease, intrahepatic growth pattern, susceptibility to chemotherapy agents and embolization, associated disabling endocrinopathies, and resectability of the primary cancers despite extensive metastases. Consequently, cytoreductive surgery is typically reserved for patients with locally advanced tumors or tumors with limited distant disease and established responsiveness to chemotherapeutic agents or radiation.

Gastrointestinal neuroendocrine malignancies are particularly well suited to cytoreductive surgery. First, survival of patients with gastrointestinal neuroendocrine tumors is widely recognized as prolonged compared to other gastrointestinal malignancies.[2] Although few studies, in fact, actually have examined the natural history of patients with gastrointestinal neuroendocrine cancers, this feature of neuroendocrine malignancies is widely accepted. Moreover, it is unknown whether the presence and type of endocrinopathy affects the natural history. Moertel et al.[3] have shown that 50% of incurable metastatic abdominal carcinoid tumors survive 5 or more years after diagnosis. Median survival of patients with unresectable hepatic metastases was greater than 3 years, and nearly 30% of these patients were alive at 5 years. Data regarding the natural history of islet cell tumors are sparse. However, Thompson et al.[4] found similar survival for patients with unresected metastatic islet cell carcinomas. Median survival of patients with hepatic metastases was 4 years, and nearly 40% were alive at 5 years after diagnosis. Clearly, the natural history of these tumors is prolonged even in patients with metastatic disease. Moreover, these patients suffer for prolonged periods of time from associated endocrinopathies.

Whether clinical endocrinopathies further affect natural history is unknown. Theoretically uncontrolled or uncontrollable endocrinopathies should affect survival adversely. Carcinoid heart disease adds cardiac failure to gastrointestinal obstruction of midgut carcinoids. Gastrinomas are predisposed to gastrointestinal perforation and hemorrhage. Insulinomas can cause hypoglycemic events leading to altered states of consciousness and subsequent morbidity and mortality. VIPomas can lead to life-threatening electrolyte abnormalities associated with incapacitating diarrhea. Durable relief of such endocrinopathies should improve survival. Norton et al.[5] have shown that patients with metastatic gastrinomas had a median survival of 3.5 years, and nearly 20% of these patients survived for 10 years. Importantly, however, the endocrinopathy was almost always controlled in these patients with H_2-receptor antagonists or H^+–K^+ ATPase inhibitors.

The clinical implication is that the therapeutic window for intervention is long and the potential to improve quality of life is great. The local growth features of the primary neuroendocrine malignancy permit resection far more frequently than other gastrointestinal malignancies of similar origin such as pancreatic ductal adenocarcinoma and small bowel adenocarcinoma. Islet cell tumors of the pancreas are often expansile in relation to the major local visceral organs or vasculature permitting resection of even large tumors. In contrast, carcinoids of the small intestine are associated with a desmoplastic reaction and can make resection of the primary tumor and the regional lymph nodes challenging but rarely precludes resection. Lastly, the severity of the endocrinopathy parallels the tumor volume. Consequently, a reduction of the bulk of the tumor mass, even when not curative, will often alleviate symptoms. Clinically, a reduction of the neuroendocrine tumor mass by complete or greater than 90% by volume has evolved as the goal for cytoreductive surgery.

The intrahepatic growth pattern of neuroendocrine metastases often permits an aggressive surgical approach. Most neuroendocrine metastases are discrete, large, and displace but do not encase the major intrahepatic vasculature or bile ducts. Such metastases can be resected or enucleated with small margins (< 1 cm) with preservation of adjacent parenchyma. From our experience, unpublished follow-up imaging data suggest that recurrences at the hepatic margins of resection are infrequent. Sclerosis of adjacent liver or adherence to intrahepatic vasculature or ducts is unusual unless preoperative arterial embolization has been performed. Some patients will have a miliary pattern of hepatic metastases with or without large dominant metastases. However, miliary metastases do not affect the resectability of larger metastases; thus given the slow tumor growth rate, resection of bulky larger metastases is reasonable for palliation. Although gastrointestinal neuroendocrine cancers can be associated with an enlarged hypervascular liver, only elevated hepatic venous pressures from cardiac failure secondary to carcinoid heart disease actually precludes resection.

Resection of the primary tumor, despite incompletely resectable metastases, is important to eliminate mechanical symptoms of the primary tumor. Primary gastrointestinal carcinoids frequently cause partial gastrointestinal obstruction or regional intestinal ischemia. Although gut carcinoids often metastasize extramurally to regional mesenteric lymph nodes, segmental enteric resection with accompanying mesentery will appropriately address the primary and regional disease. Mesenteric adenopathy, though bulky, usually displaces major mesenteric vessels to the periphery of the mesenteric mass which permits preservation of the gut vasculature. Similarly, islet cell cancers seldom encase the celiac or superior mesenteric arteries or the portal venous system. Distal islet cell cancers, however, often invade the splenic vein or spleen. This may lead to sinistral hypertension and gastric variceal bleeding. Resection of the primary pancreatic tumor is the treatment of choice for this type of gastric bleeding.

3.   PATIENTS AND METHODS

The data analyzed in this report were accrued through a review of the English language medical literature from January 1973 to April 1999. Reports of hepatic resection for metastatic neuroendocrine malignancies were culled. The gastrointestinal neuroendocrine malignancies were stratified into two basic groups of analysis: carcinoid and noncarcinoid neuroendocrine malignancies. The latter group was composed predominantly of functioning islet cell carcinomas. Factors related to the patients and operative procedures, which were abstracted from the reports, included number of patients, resection of the primary tumor, type of hepatic resection, extent of cytoreductive procedure (partial or total gross resection), operative morbidity and mortality for the cytoreductive procedure, duration of survival, duration of clinical response, degree of clinical response (none, partial, or complete), and adjuvant or adjunctive chemotherapy. Factors related to the tumor which were abstracted from the literature review included: presence or absence of clinical endocrinopathy, type of endocrinopathy, type and level of serum hormonal markers, extent of hepatic metastases, extent (stage) of primary tumor, objective response to cytoreduction by hormonal marker level or body imaging, and pattern of disease recurrence. Cumulative survival for patients with both carcinoid and noncarcinoid neuroendocrine malignancies were estimated by the Kaplan–Meier method based upon the duration of survival specified for each patient in each report included within our review. Statistical analyses of patient- and tumor-related factors to survival were precluded due to the small number of patients in this review and the variability in reporting. Our recent report[6] was excluded from the analysis of the literature to reduce bias in outcome because our experience exceeded that cumulatively compiled herein.

4.   LITERATURE REVIEW

4.1.   Endocrinopathies

Cytoreductive hepatic surgery for metastatic carcinoid disease was performed in 164 patients (Table 1). Of these, 109 patients had symptoms of the carcinoid syndrome

Table 1. The outcome of partial hepatectomy in patients for metastatic carcinoid and islet cell cancers—literature review

References	Carcinoid	Noncarcinoid	Endocrine symptoms	Clinical response	Recurrence	Operative mortality	Survival (month)
Stephen[21]	5	–	5	5	0	0	12–30
Davis[22]	2	–	2	NR	1	0	18–30
Battersby[23]	1	–	1	1	1 (re-resected)	0	22
Fotner[24]	2	–	NR	NR	0	1	0–9
Gillett[25]	2	–	2	2	0	0	12
Kune[26]	1	–	1	1	1	0	7
Lannon[27]	1	–	1	1	1	0	8
Longmire[28]	1	–	1	NR	0	1	0
Reiss[29]	2	–	0	NR	1	0	36–96
Aronsen[30]	1	–	1	1	1	–	96
Foster[31]	7	–	7	6	5	1	7–120
Taylor[32]	1	–	1	NR	1	0	46
Thompson[33]	1	–	NR	NR	NR	0	47
Norton[34]	–	3	3	3	1	0	18–32
Stehlin[35]	4	–	NR	NR	4	0	8–172
Akerstrom[36]	1	–	1	1	0	0	36
Wolf[37]	2	–	NR	NR	0	0	16–26
	–	2	NR	NR	1	0	11–27
Dousset[38]	10	–	6	6	6	0	6–36
	7		3	3	4 (2 re-resected)	1	0.3–108
Berney[39]	–	1	NR	NR	0	0	22
Sarmiento (unpublished data)	120	50	108	104	99	2	81 (median)

NR = not reported.
Data cited refer to number of patients.

and 33 patients had clinically evident valvular right heart disease. Specific symptoms and signs as a clinical presentation, such as flushing, diarrhea, wheezing, etc., were not detailed sufficiently to determine overall frequency. The preoperative duration of carcinoid tumor-related symptoms before cytoreduction ranged from a few weeks to 11 years. Urinary 5-hydroxyindoleacetic acid (5-HIAA) values were elevated in every patient in whom levels were obtained. Primary carcinoids arose from the small intestine in 52% of patients. The other primary carcinoids arose from the lung in 4% of patients and were unknown in the remaining patients (ovary, pancreas, and appendix in one patient each). The primary site was not reported in 13 of the 164 patients. Cytoreductive hepatic surgery for metastatic islet cell tumors was performed in 63 patients (Table 1). Twenty-four (38%) of the patients with metastatic noncarcinoid gastrointestinal neuroendocrine cancers had endocrinopathies from excess hormone production. The severity of the clinical endocrinopathy was attributed to metastatic disease or overall tumor burden in each report. Clinical endocrinopathies varied depending upon the hormone produced by the malignancy. There were 14 gastrinomas, 3 VIPomas, 10 glucagonoma, 23 nonfunctioning APUDomas, and 7 insulinomas. Eleven patients had overproduction of multiple hormones. In patients with multiple hormone production, only one hormone caused a clinical endocrinopathy, and symptoms of that endocrinopathy did not differ clinically from descriptions of that specific islet cell endocrine syndrome, i.e. other hormones did not affect clinical presentation. Only five patients had cytoreduction for nonfunctioning islet cell malignancies and in all of them in our own series. The duration of endocrine symptoms prior to hepatectomy ranged from 18 to 42 months. Most patients had prior therapy in an attempt to control endocrinopathies either by resection of the primary tumor, chemotherapy, or pharmacologic agents. The series at Mayo, however, contains patients in who surgery was the primary therapy in 62%. Hormone markers for each endocrinopathy were obtained in most patients and were pathologically elevated in nearly all of these patients.

Orthotopic liver transplantation for metastatic neuroendocrine cancers was performed in 92 patients (Table 2). Of these, 43% patients had metastatic carcinoids, 43% had metastatic islet cell cancers, and 14% had tumors classified only as neuroendocrine. Symptomatic endocrinopathies were present in 49% of patients. Carcinoids originated from the small intestine in 17, lung in 8, and other sites in 15. Islet cell cancers included 9 gastrinomas, 4 glucagonomas, 2 VIPomas, 2 GHRFomas, 1 insulinoma, 1 parathyroid hormone-related peptide, and 15 nonfunctioning cancers. Five patients had overproduction of multiple hormones and 13 were unknown or not reported. The primary neuroendocrine cancer was resected prior to orthotopic liver transplantation in 29% of patients, concurrently in 28%, and was not stated or unknown in 38% of patients. Four patients' primary tumor was found and resected after orthotopic liver transplantation.

5. EXTENT OF NEUROENDOCRINE MALIGNANCIES

Primary carcinoid tumors had been previously resected from 0.7 to 72 months previously in six patients. Most of the reported resections were synchronous (76 patients). Stage of the primary carcinoid could not be determined from the literature. Hepatic metastases were multiple in the majority of patients but a specific number of metastases could not

Table 2. The outcome of orthotopic liver transplantation in patients with metastatic carcinoid and islet cell cancers—literature review

References	Carcinoid	Noncarcinoid	Not reported	Recurrence	Operative mortality	Survival (month)
O'Grady[40]	2	–	–	1	0	7–12
Makowka[41]	2	–	–	0	1 (re: OLT)	2–9
	–	3	–	1	0	10–160
Ringe[42]	2	–	–	1	1	0.3–6
	–	1	–	0	0	5
Alsina[43]	1	1	–	0	0	13
	–	1	–	0	0	5
Gulaniker[44]	1	–	–	0	0	5
Lobe[45]	–	1	–	0	0	15
Farmer[46]	2	–	–	0	0	22–29
Schweizer[47]	–	1	–	1	0	10
Bechstein[48]	1	–	–	1	0	42
Frilling[49]	1	–	–	0	0	10
Alessiani[50]	–	–	9	3	0	17–61
Curtiss[51]	–	3	–	0	0	12–30
Routley[52]	6	–	–	4	0	8–67
	–	5	–	1	0	8–106
Anthuber[53]	2	–	–	1	1	0.3–4
	–	1	–	1	0	15
Dousset[38]	4	–	–	1	1 (re: OLT)	0.2–62
	–	5	–	1	3 (2 re: OLT)	0.2–17
Lang[54]	3	–	–	–	1	0.4–58
	–	5	–	2	0	47–103.5
	–	–	4	3	0	2–70
Le Treut[55]	11	–	–	6 (1 re-resected)	0	2–77
	–	12	–	7	3	0.2–51
Caplin[56]	1	–	–	1	0	15
Hengst[57]	–	1	–	0	0	20
Savelli[58]	1	–	–	1	0	32

Data cited refer to number of patients.

be tabulated because of data presentation. Hepatic carcinoid metastases range from 0.8 to 15 cm in greatest diameter. Few patients had concurrent extrahepatic, intra-abdominal disease excluding the primary tumor. The primary islet cell carcinomas have been resected previously in five patients and synchronously in 35 patients. As with carcinoid tumors, stage of the primary tumors at initial diagnosis could not be determined.

5.1. Resection of Metastatic Neuroendocrine Malignancy

Partial hepatectomy for metastatic neuroendocrine malignancies (both carcinoid and noncarcinoid) was performed overall in 227 patients and total hepatectomy with orthotopic liver transplantation was performed in 92 patients. Types of partial hepatectomy was reported for 212 patients included hemihepatectomy in 96 (45%) patients, wedge resection in 34 (16%) patients, extended lobar resections (i.e. right or left hepatectomy with either contiguous or noncontiguous resection of contralateral metastases) in 30 (14%) patients, and enucleation in 2 (5%) patients. Five additional patients had an undefined type of major hepatic resection. The rest of the patients had resection of one to three segments of the liver.

5.2. Morbidity and Mortality

Overall morbidity for cytoreductive hepatic surgery was 14% (29 of 212 patients). Operative mortality after partial hepatectomy for metastatic carcinoid disease was 2.3% (5 of 212 patients). Excluding perioperative deaths, complications directly related to cytoreductive hepatic surgery for carcinoid tumors included postoperative liver failure in one patient and liver failure, pulmonary embolus, pleural effusion, and small bowel obstruction in another patient.

Operative mortality for hepatic resection for metastatic islet cell carcinomas was 1.6% (1 of 63 patients). Major postoperative morbidity for metastatic islet cell carcinoma included subdiaphragmatic bile collection, intra-abdominal hemorrhage, and subdiaphragmatic abscess. Other reported morbidity for cytoreductive hepatic surgery included biliary fistula in two patients, pancreatic fistula in two patients, and infected hematoma in two patients.

There were 11 postoperative deaths following a total hepatectomy and orthotopic liver transplantation for metastatic neuroendocrine tumors. Death was attributed to irreversible rejection after two orthotopic liver transplantations in one patient, cardiac failure in two patients, sepsis in three patients, persistent intra-abdominal hemorrhage in five patients—associated with acute pancreatitis in two patients, thrombosis of the portal vein in two patients, and primary nonfunctioning in one patient. Five patients required retransplantation; three for chronic rejection, one for portal vein thrombosis, and one for primary nonfunction. Four of the five suffered operative deaths.

5.3. Survival After Cytoreductive Hepatic Surgery

The overall survival of patients with metastatic neuroendocrine tumors after partial hepatectomy and following cytoreductive partial hepatectomy for malignant carcinoid tumors is discussed here. Median survival could not be estimated due to the limited duration of follow-up among reports. The relationship of survival to number of metastases, margins of resection, or type of resection could not be established from the literature review. Only 43 carcinoid patients had no evidence of disease recurrence with the limits of follow-up ranging from 4 to 36 months. Four additional patients had repeat resection of recurrent disease and remained without evidence of disease recurrence. Median survival could not be estimated with currently available follow-up data. There was no difference in survival after hepatic resection by type of endocrinopathy. The malignant gastrinomas and nonfunctioning APUDomas were the most common malignancy among these patients, but these tumors were the most prevalent tumors reported. Ten patients had no evidence of disease recurrence with limited duration of follow-up. Two patients had resection of recurrent tumor at 12 and 16 months, respectively, and remained without evidence of disease recurrence at 60 and 108 months, respectively.

Survival for carcinoid tumors was 44% at 5 years with a median survival of 3.4 years. Survival for noncarcinoid neuroendocrine cancers was 43% at 5 years. Recurrence was reported in 38 patients. Death was attributed to recurrence of neuroendocrine tumor in 15 patients after liver transplantation. Recurrence was reported in the liver in 7 patients, in bone in 11, in lung in 3, and mesenteric lymph nodes in 3. One other patient had recurrence of a cholangiocarcinoma, which was diagnosed after transplantation for a neuroendocrine tumor. Death was attributed to recurrent cholangiocarcinoma.

5.4.   Symptomatic Response

Symptomatic response of carcinoid syndrome resolved completely in 86% of patients undergoing partial cytoreductive hepatectomy. The duration of complete response from carcinoid syndrome ranged from 4 to 120 months. Forty-one patients had no recurrence of symptoms or objective disease (i.e. normal 5-HIAA values and the absence of metastasis on imaging studies). Relationship between the onset and severity of recurrent symptoms and the extent of disease recurrence based on either 5-HIAA values or imaging studies could not be determined in this review. Clinical response to cytoreduction was incomplete in three patients. The duration of incomplete response could not be estimated from the literature data. Excluding operative deaths, only one patient selected for cytoreductive surgery failed to respond clinically.[7] Objective measurements of response to cytoreductive hepatic surgery by either 5-HIAA values or body imaging modalities were limited. In general, 5-HIAA levels were reduced following resection. However, further quantitation of 5-HIAA response was precluded because of assay variability. The mean duration of complete objective response from these patients could not be estimated because of insufficient data. Due to the time period of this literature review, summary of objective imaging follow-up for recurrent disease was also precluded.

Symptomatic response of islet cell tumor endocrinopathies resolved completely in all three patients for whom clinical response was reported. Clinical response was not stated for three patients and the extent of response was not stated for two patients that responded. Twenty-three patients had nonfunctioning tumors. The duration of complete symptom-free response from the endocrinopathies could not be determined. Seventeen patients had no recurrence by hormonal markers or objective imaging studies. Similar to carcinoid patients, the relationship of hormonal marker values and the onset in severity of recurrent symptoms could not be determined. Although comparison of responses after partial or complete resection is relative, reports suggest a greater degree and duration of benefit for complete resection of the metastatic disease and control of the primary tumor than for partial resection. Of those patients with endocrinopathies persisting after resection, reduction of hormone values was documented in two of three patients. Hormonal response was not detailed in one patient. Meaningful analysis of "disease-free" survival based on imaging data was precluded because of the variety of abdominal imaging used in follow-up and the lack of uniform frequency of follow-up imaging.

No patient following orthotopic liver transplantation failed to respond clinically. Correlation of objective measurements of response to total hepatectomy by serum hormone values or body imaging modalities expectedly paralleled clinical response. Biochemical recurrence without clinical recurrence developed in two patients following liver transplantation.

5.5.   Adjuvant and Adjunctive Therapy

Sixty-five patients had adjunctive therapy. Three patients had a single recurrent hepatic nodule successfully treated by percutaneous alcohol injection. Twenty-one patients were treated with cytoreductive chemotherapy; five patients underwent intra-arterial chemoembolization. Data are too heterogeneous to allow a proper analysis of this subset of patients.

5.6.   Cryotherapy

Hepatic cryosurgery is a widely used and well-recognized modality for treatment of hepatic tumors. Cozzi et al.[8] demonstrated for the first time that hepatic cryotherapy offered adjunctive treatment for patients with neuroendocrine hepatic tumors. All six patients had a complete radiologic response, remain alive and asymptomatic with a median follow-up of 24 months. There was also an 89% decrease in elevated tumor markers. Bilchik et al.[9] showed that cryosurgery dramatically relieved symptoms with a significant reduction in tumor markers. The median symptom-free and overall survivals were 10 months and more than 49 months, respectively. While hepatic cryotherapy is feasible in the treatment of neuroendocrine liver metastases, its role as an alternative to liver resection is not yet well supported by long-term data. Other techniques of local tumor ablation including radio frequency ablation, percutaneous microwave coagulation, laser interstitial photocoagulation, and carbon dioxide laser, although promising, remain unproved. Currently, we used radio frequency ablation in conjunction with metastasectomy to maximally preserve functional hepatic parenchyma.

6.   CONCLUSIONS

This review suggests that cytoreductive hepatic resection for functioning metastatic neuroendocrine malignancies was efficacious in selected patients. Resection of hepatic metastases promptly relieved clinical endocrinopathies in nearly all patients and symptomatic response often lasted many months. Perioperative morbidity and mortality was limited. Moreover, current data support further investigation of the role of hepatic transplantation in patients with isolated hepatic metastases from gastrointestinal neuroendocrine cancers. Current data confirm that hepatic resection, either concurrent with or subsequent to resection of the primary gastrointestinal neuroendocrine cancer, is safe.

Our own experience and that reported in this review have shown that cytoreductive surgery is safe.[6] Admittedly, patient selection was careful, and publication bias may favor a positive patient outcome. We previously reported on operative mortality of 2.7% and operative morbidity of 24%, which does not differ from this literature review. Our overall symptomatic response rate was 90% with a mean duration of 19.3 months. Patient selection clearly influenced outcome. Reports to date may be biased toward a positive clinical response and low perioperative mortality and morbidity. Regardless of this potential, however, greater than 85% of the patients had major hepatic resections (hemi- or extended hemihepatectomy) and more than 40% of the patients had concurrent resection of the primary gastrointestinal neuroendocrine cancer. The fact that these collective data do not differ from the perioperative risk for major hepatic resections for other metastatic cancers and are less than the risk for resection of primary hepatic malignancies with cirrhosis supports hepatic cytoreduction for these tumors. Specific endocrinopathies have not increased perioperative risk with the possible exception of carcinoid heart disease. Operative repair of carcinoid heart disease may be required prior to hepatic resection for symptomatic carcinoid syndrome in very selected patients to reduce the risk of massive hemorrhage caused by intrahepatic venous hypertension from right heart failure.[10] Finally, clinical response rates from the compiled literature were similar to our own experience.[6] Durability of responses could not be quantitated from the list; however, our data confirmed a mean duration of response for nearly 20 months before subsequent therapy was undertaken.

Orthotopic liver transplantation for metastatic neuroendocrine cancers has been employed more frequently since our prior report. These tumors have become the primary indication for transplantation for metastatic disease. Although current results confirm that hepatic transplantation is uniformly effective for symptomatic relief, current survival data herein raise concerns over the appropriateness of such therapy for carcinoid tumors. Another independent review of 103 patients who underwent hepatic transplantation for metastatic neuroendocrine cancers found an overall 5-year survival of 47%, but a recurrene-free 5-year survival of only 24%.[11] Perioperative mortality was 10%. Multivariate analysis showed that age greater than 50 years and transplantation with upper abdominal exenteration or Whipple's operation as adverse prognostic factors. Perhaps more accurate preoperative staging with octreotide scanning and MR will permit better patient selection for hepatic transplantation. Nonetheless, if future socioeconomic factors and organ availability permit hepatic transplantation in patients with metastatic cancer, this option for improved quality of life in these previously end-stage patients with neuroendocrine cancers may be more widely accepted.

There is no consensus on adjunctive chemotherapy or biotherapy for patients with malignant neuroendocrine tumors. These therapies are usually reserved for patients with advanced, inoperable, or residual disease. In practice, chemotherapy is usually withheld until all surgical options are exhausted. Combination chemotherapy with streptozotocin and 5-fluorouracil or doxorubicin is still considered the first-line treatment for malignant neuroendocrine tumors.[12–14] The majority of patients treated had metastatic carcinoid tumor and, in general, the outcome has been disappointing.[15,16] However, in patients with predominantly anaplastic neuroendocrine tumors in advanced stages, good tumor response rates with a combination of cisplatin and etoposide can be achieved.[17]

Neuroendocrine gastrointestinal tumors express somatostatin receptors in 80–90% of patients, and somatostatin analogs have become important in the treatment of those patients. Although objective tumor regression occurs in only 10–20% of patients, stabilization of tumor growth is achieved in nearly half of the patients with a duration of 8–16 months.[18] Interferon-alpha has been used as an alternative to somatostatin analogs. A median biochemical response rate of 44% and a tumor response rate of 11% have been observed.[19] The current medical treatment of neuroendocrine tumors is based on chemotherapy for more highly proliferating tumors, such as malignant endocrine pancreatic tumors and foregut carcinoids, while biotherapy, including interferon-alpha and somatostatin analogs, is used in slow-growing tumors such as midgut carcinoids.[13]

Clear guidelines for patient selection are evolving. In general, if both the primary neuroendocrine cancer and its regional and hepatic metastases are resectable based on preoperative imaging studies, exploration for resection is clearly the treatment of choice. Conversely, if neither the local extent of the primary and regional neuroendocrine cancer or its hepatic metastasis is resectable, medical treatment is advised. Most patients, however, present clinically between these extremes. Indeed, most patients will have resectable primary tumors but incompletely resectable or ablatable hepatic metastases. If hepatic metastases are multiple and bilobar, the decision for cytoreductive surgery is more complex. In general, if an expected 90% or greater of the hepatic disease can be removed with the primary and regional disease, then exploration is advised. If less than 90% of the hepatic metastases with the primary tumor are resectable or ablatable, then cytoreductive surgery is currently not indicated because the duration and degree of symptomatic response following such surgery is expectedly brief. However, if effective adjunctive treatments become available, cytoreduction to a lesser degree may become indicated.

Accurate imaging is essential for evaluating potential candidates with neuroendocrine carcinoma for hepatic resection. In general, MRI with contrast enhancement is the single most accurate imaging modality for hepatic metastases from neuroendocrine tumors. MR accurately and clearly defines these hypervascular metastases and their relationship to the intrahepatic vasculature. Moreover, MR cholangiography can be obtained concurrently if indicated. Imaging of the primary tumor depends on the site of origin with enteroclysis best for carcinoid tumors and rapid contrast enhanced CT for most islet cell carcinomas. Whether octreotide scanning should be routinely employed in all patients with metastatic neuroendocrine carcinomas is unknown. To date, most reports addressing cytoreductive hepatic surgery have not employed octreotide scanning as an option for resection. Although imaging of patients with metastatic neuroendocrine carcinomas with octreotide scanning probably would have a high positivity rate, the responses to date obtained after cytoreductive surgery without octreotide scanning would question its necessity because treatment is primarily palliative. Perhaps octreotide scanning should be routinely used in patients prior to hepatic transplantation given the socioeconomic impact of this therapy.

Perioperative preparation of patients with neuroendocrine carcinoma is similar to that for patients for other hepatic malignancies, except for control of the endocrinopathy preoperatively is important. Our data have shown that for patients with malignant carcinoid tumors, preoperative antihormonal therapy with a somatostatin analog is essential to prevent carcinoid crisis at the time of resection. Preoperative preparation with 150–500 µg of somatostatin on call to the operating room prevents hemodynamic instability intraoperatively.[20] Similarly, control of other neuroendocrine tumors with adequate glucose monitoring for insulinomas and H_2-receptor antagonists or H^+–K^+ ATPase inhibitors for gastrinomas are essential.

Hepatic resection for metastatic neuroendocrine tumors is done primarily for palliative purposes. The intent of surgery is to resect or ablate 90% or greater of the hepatic
disease. Consequently, ablative technology [cytoablative or thermal (microwave or radio
frequency) units] should be available for adjunctive intraoperative use. Hepatic tumors are
approached as any metastatic tumor with the intent to resect all gross tumor with a tumor-free
margin. All bulky disease is resected or ablated. Cholecystectomy is routinely performed
to eliminate potential complications from future hepatic arterial embolization or use of
somatostatin analogs. Regional lymphadenectomy of the hepatoduodenal ligament, portal
vein, and hepatic and celiac arteries is performed for all islet cell cancers and selected
carcinoids. Excision of gross nodal disease during partial hepatectomy will ensure optimal long-term hepatic blood flow and reduce the risk of subsequent extrahepatic bile duct
obstruction.

REFERENCES

1. Wong WJ, DeCosse JJ. Cytoreductive surgery. *Surg Gynecol Obstet.* 1990;170:276–281.
2. Moertel CG. An odyssey in the land of small tumors. *J Clin Oncol.* 1987;5:1503–1522.
3. Moertel CG, Sauer WG, Dockerty MB, Baggenstoss AH. Life history of the carcinoid tumor of the small intestine. *Cancer.* 1961;14:901–912.
4. Thompson GB, van Heerden JA, Grant CS, Carney JA, Ilstrup DM. Iset cell carcinoma of the pancreas: a twenty year experience. *Surgery.* 1988;104:1011–1017.
5. Norton JA, Doppman JL, Jensen RT. Curative resection in Zollinger-Ellison syndrome. Results of a 10-year prospective study. *Ann Surg.* 1992;215:8–18.
6. Que FG, Nagorney DM, Batts KP, Linz LJ, Kvols LK. Hepatic resection for metastatic neuroendocrine carcinomas. *Am J Surg.* 1995;169:36.
7. McEntee GP, Nagorney DM, Kvols LK, Moertel CG, Grant CS. Cytoreductive hepatic surgery for neuroen-docrine tumors. *Surgery.* 1990;108:1091–1096.
8. Cozzi PJ, England R, Morris DL. Cryotherapy treatment of patients with hepatic metastases from neuroen-docrine tumors. *Cancer.* 1995;76:501–509.
9. Bilchik AJ, Sarantou T, Foshag LJ, Giuliano AE, Ramming KP. Cryosurgical palliation of metastatic neuroen-docrine tumors resistant to conventional therapy. *Surgery.* 1997;122:1040–1047.
10. McDonald ML, Nagorney DM, Connolly HM, Nisimura RA, Schaff HV. Carcinoid heart disease and carcinoid syndrome: successful surgical treatment. *Ann Thorac Surg.* 1999;67:537–539.
11. Lehnert T. Liver transplantation for metastatic neuroendocrine carcinoma. *Transplantation.* 1998;66:1307–1312.
12. Kelsen DG, Cheng E, Kemeny H. Streptozotocin and adriamycin in the treatment of APUD tumors. *Proc Am Assoc Cancer Res.* 1982;23:433.
13. Oberg K. Advances in chemotherapy and biotherapy of endocrine tumors. *Curr Opin.* 1998;10:58–65.
14. Moertel CG, Lefkopoulo M, Lipsitz S, Hahn RG, Klaassen D. Streptozocin-doxorubicin, streptozocin-fluorouracil or chlorozotocin in the treatment of advanced islet-cell carcinoma. *N Engl J Med.* 1992;326:519–523.
15. Kvols LK. Therapy of malignant carcinoid syndrome. *Endocrinol Metab Clin North Am.* 1989;18:557–568.
16. Moertel CG, Johnson CM, McKusick MA, et al. The management of patients with advanced carcinoid tumors and islet cell carcinomas. *Ann Intern Med.* 1994;120:302–309.
17. Moertel CG, Kvols LK, O'Connell MJ, Rubin J. Treatment of neuroendocrine carcinomas with combined etoposide and cisplatin. Evidence of major therapeutic activity in the anaplastic variants of these neoplasms. *Cancer.* 1991;68:227–232.
18. Eriksson B, Oberg K. Summing up 15 years of somatostatin analog therapy in neuroendocrine tumors: future outlook. *Ann Oncol.* 1999;10:531–538.

19. Oberg K. Interferon-alpha versus somatostatin or the combination of both in gastroenteropancreatic tumors. *Digestion.* 1996;57:83.
20. Kinney MA, Warner ME, Nagorney DM, Rubin J, Schroeder DR, Maxson PM, Warner MA. Perianaesthetic risk and outcomes of abdominal surgery for metastatic carcinoid tumours. *Br J Anaesth.* 2001 Sep;87(3):497–452.
21. Stephen JL, Grahame-Smith jDG. Treatment of the carcinoid syndrome by local removal of hepatic metastases. *Proc R Soc Med.* 1972;65:444–445.
22. Davis Z, Moertel CG, McIlrath DC. The malignant carcinoid syndrome. *Surg Gynecol Obstet.* 1973;137:637–644.
23. Battersby C, Egerton WS. A carcinoid saga. *ANZ J Surg.* 1974;44:32–84.
24. Fotner JG, Kinne DW, Kim DK, Castro EB, Shiu MH, Beattie EJJ. Vascular problems in upper abdominal cancer surgery. *Arch Surg.* 1974;109:148–153.
25. Gillett DJ, Smith RC. Treatment of the carcinoid syndrome by hemihepatectomy and radical excision of primary lesion. *Am J Surg.* 1974;128:95–99.
26. Kune GA, Goldstein J. Malignant liver carcinoid: the place of surgery and chemotherapy. Review and case presentation. *Med J Aust.* 1974;2:777–780.
27. Lannon J. Seventeen cases of hepatectomy. *S Afr J Surg.* 1974;12:227–232.
28. Longmire WPJ, Trout HHd, Greenfield J, Tompkins RK. Elective hepatic surgery. *Ann Surg.* 1974;179:712–721.
29. Reiss R, Antal SC. Indications for partial hepatectomy in metastatic disease. *Bull Soc Int Chir.* 1974;33:172–177.
30. Aronsen KF, Torp A, Waldenstrom JG. A case of carcinoid syndrome followed for eight years after palliative liver resection. *Acta Med Scand.* 1976;199:327–329.
31. Foster JH, Berman MM. Palliative liver resection to relieve symptoms of the malignant carcinoid and other endocrine syndromes. *Solid Liver Tumors.* Vol. 22. Philadelphia: W. B. Saunders Company 1977;235–245.
32. Taylor B, Langer B, Falk RE, Ambus U. Role of resection in the management of metastases to the liver. *Can J Surg.* 1983;26:215–217.
33. Thompson HH, Tompkins RK, Longmire WPJ. Major hepatic resection: a 25-year experience. *Ann Surg.* 1983;197:375–387.
34. Norton JA, Sugarbaker PH, Doppman JL, et al. Aggressive resection of metastatic disease in selected patients with malignant gastrinoma. *Ann Surg.* 1986;203:352–359.
35. Stehlin JS, Jr., De Ipoly PD, Greeff PJ, McGaff CJ, Jr., Davis BR, McNary L. Treatment of cancer of the liver. Twenty years' experience with infusion and resection in 414 patients. *Ann Surg.* 1988;208:23–35.
36. Akerstrom G, Makridis C, Johansson H. Abdominal surgery in patients with midgut carcinoid tumors. *Acta Oncol.* 1991;30:547–553.
37. Wolf RF, Goodnight JE, Krag DE, Schneider PD. Results of resection and proposed guidelines for patient selection in instances of noncolorectal hepatic metastases. *Surg Gynecol Obstet.* 1991;173:454–460.
38. Dousset B, Saint-Marc O, Pitre J, Sourbrane O, Houssin D, Chapuis Y. Metastatic endocrine tumors: medical treatment, surgical resection, or liver transplantation. *World J Surg.* 1996;20:908–915.
39. Berney T, Mentha G, Roth AD, Morel P. Results of surgical resection of liver metastasis from non-colorectal primaries. *Br J Surg.* 1998;85:1423–1427.
40. O'Grady JG, Polson RJ, Rolles K, Calne RY, Williams R. Liver transplantation for malignant disease. Results in 93 consecutive patients. *Ann Surg.* 1988;207:373–379.
41. Makowka L, Tzakis AG, Mazzaferro V, et al. Transplantation of the liver for metastatic neuroendocrine tumors of the intestine and pancreas. *Surg Gynecol Obstet.* 1989;168:107–111.
42. Ringe B, Wittekind C, Bechstein WO, Bunzendahl H, Pichlmayr R. The role of liver transplantation in hepatobiliary malignancy. A retrospective analysis of 95 patients with particular regard to tumor stage and recurrence. *Ann Surg.* 1989;209:88–98.
43. Alsina AE, Bartus S, Hull D, Rosson R, Schweizer RT. Liver transplant for metastatic neuroendocrine tumor. *J Clin Gastroenterol.* 1990;12:533–537.
44. Gulanikar AC, Kotylak G, Bitter-Suermann H. Does immunosuppression alter the growth of metastatic liver carcinoid after orthotopic liver transplantation? *Transplant Proc.* 1991;23:2197–2198.

45. Lobe TE, Vera SR, Bowman LC, Fontanesi J, Britt LG, Gaber AO. Hepaticopancreatidcogastroduodenectomy with transplantation for metastatic islet cell carcinoma in childhood. *J Pediatr Surg.* 1992;27:227–229.
46. Farmer DG, Shaked A, Colonna JOI, et al. Radical resection combined with liver transplantation for foregut tumors. *Am Surg.* 1993;59:806–812.
47. Schweizer RT, Alsina AE, Rosson R, Bartus SA. Liver transplantation for metastatic neuroendocrine tumors. *Transplant Proc.* 1993;25:1973.
48. Bechstein WO, Neuhaus P. Liver transplantation for hepatic metastases of neuroendocrine tumors. *Ann N Y Acad Sci.* 1994;733:507–514.
49. Frilling A, Rogiers X, Knofel WT, Broelsch CE. Liver transplantation for metastatic carcinoid tumors. *Digestion.* 1994;55:104–106.
50. Alessiani M, Tzakis A, Todo S, Demetris AJ, Fung JJ, Starzl TE. Assessment of five-year experience with abdominal organ cluster transplantation. *J Am Coll Surg.* 1995;180:1–9.
51. Curtiss SI, Mor E, Schwartz ME, et al. The rational approach to the use of hepatic transplantation in the treatment of metastatic neuroendocrine tumors. *J Am Coll Surg.* 1995;180:184–187.
52. Routley D, Ramage JK, McPeake J, Tan K-C, Williams R. Orthotopic liver transplantation in the treatment of metastatic neuroendocrine tumors of the liver. *Liver Transplant Surg.* 1995;1:118–121.
53. Anthuber M, Jauch KW, Briegel J, Groh J, Schildberg FW. Results of liver transplantation for gastroenteropancreatic tumor metastases. *World J Surg.* 1996;20:73–76.
54. Lang H, Oldhafer KJ, Weimann A, et al. Liver transplantation for metastatic neuroendocrine tumors. *Ann Surg.* 1997;225:347–354.
55. Le Treut YP, Delpero JR, Dousset B, et al. Results of liver transplantation in the treatment of metastatic neuroendocrine tumors. A 31-case French multicentric report. *Ann Surg.* 1997;225:355–364.
56. Caplin ME, Hodgson HJ, Dhillon AP, et al. Multimodality treatment for gastric carcinoid tumor with liver metastasis. *Am J Gastroenterol.* 1998;93:1945–1948.
57. Hengst K, Nashan B, Avenhaus W, et al. Metastatic pancreatic VIPoma: Deteriorating clinical course and successful treatment by liver transplantation. *Z Gastroenterol.* 1998;36:239–245.
58. Savelli G, Chiti A, Spinelli A, et al. Bone lesion in a patient with transplanted liver for a metastatic carcinoid. The role of somatostatin receptor scintigraphy. *Tumori.* 1998;84:82–84.

Electrodes and Multiple Electrode Systems for Radio Frequency Ablation: A Proposal for Updated Terminology

STEFAAN MULIER,[*,††] YI MIAO,[†] PETER MULIER,[‡] BENOIT DUPAS,[§] PHILIPPE PEREIRA,[‖] THIERRY DE BAERE,[¶] RICCARDO LENCIONI,[#] RAYMOND LEVEILLEE,[**] GUY MARCHAL,[††] LUC MICHEL,[*] and YICHENG NI[††]

[*]Department of Surgery, University Hospital of Mont-Godinne, Catholic University of Louvain, Yvoir, Belgium; [†]Department of General Surgery, The First Affiliated Hospital of Nanjing Medical University, Nanjing, China; [‡]Biomedical engineer, Minneapolis, Minnesota, USA; [§]Department of Radiology, University Hospital of Nantes, Nantes, France; [‖]Department of Diagnostic Radiology, Eberhard-Karls-Universität Tübingen, Tübingen, Germany; [¶]Department of Radiology, Institut Gustave Roussy, Villejuif, France; [#]Division of Diagnostic and Interventional Radiology, University of Pisa, Pisa, Italy; [**]Division of Endourology, Laparoscopy and Minimally Invasive Surgery, University of Miami School of Medicine, Miami, Florida, USA; [††]Department of Radiology, University Hospital Gasthuisberg, Catholic University of Leuven, Leuven, Belgium

ABSTRACT

Objective

Research on technology for soft tissue radio frequency (RF) ablation is ever advancing. A recent proposal to standardize terminology of RF electrodes only deals with the most frequently used commercial electrodes. The aim of this study was to develop a logical, versatile, and unequivocal terminology to describe present and future RF electrodes and multiple electrode systems.

Materials and Methods

We have carried out a PubMed search for the period from January 1st 1990 to July 1st 2004 in seven languages and contacted the six major companies that produce commercial RF electrodes for use in the liver. In a first step, names have been defined for the five existing *basic designs* of single-shaft electrode. These names had to be unequivocal, descriptive of the electrode's main working principle and as short as possible. In a second step, these basic names have been used as building blocks to describe the single-shaft electrodes in *combination designs*. In a third step, using the same principles, a logical terminology has been developed for *multiple electrode systems*, defined as the combined use of more than one single-shaft RF electrode.

N. A. Habib and R. Canelo (eds.), Liver and Pancreatic Diseases Management, 57–73.
© 2006 *Springer. Printed in The Netherlands.*

Results

Five basic electrode designs were identified and defined: plain, cooled, expandable, wet, and bipolar electrodes.

Combination designs included cooled-wet, expandable-wet, bipolar-wet, bipolar-cooled, bipolar-expandable, and bipolar-cooled-wet electrodes.

Multiple electrode systems could be characterized by describing several features: the number of electrodes that were used (dual, triple, etc), the electric mode (monopolar or bipolar), the activation mode (consecutive, simultaneous or switching), the site of the inserted electrodes (monofocal or multifocal), and the type of single-shaft electrodes that were used.

Conclusion

In this terminology, the naming of the basic electrode designs has been based on objective criteria. The short and unequivocal names of the basic designs can easily be combined to describe current and future combination electrodes. This terminology provides an exact and complete description of the versatile novel multiple electrode systems.

Key words: Radio frequency ablation, Liver, Kidney, Soft tissues

1.   INTRODUCTION

The development of novel and ingenious electrodes for soft tissue (such as liver and kidney) radio frequency ablation (RFA) is expanding rapidly. Multiple names to describe RF electrodes are being utilized. A proposal to address this semantic confusion was recently published by the IWGIGTA (International Working Group on Image-Guided Tumor Ablation).[1] It described most of the commercial electrodes that were available at that moment. Since this publication, many new commercial and experimental electrodes, as well as several "multiple electrode systems" have been introduced.

The aim of this article is to update the existing classification and to present a logical and easily adoptable terminology for the generic classification of all RF electrodes and multiple electrode systems.

2.   MATERIALS AND METHODS

We carried out a PubMed search of the world literature for the period from January 1st 1990 to July 1st 2004 using the keywords (radiofrequency, radio-frequency or radio frequency) and (liver or hepatic or hepatocellular) on articles written in English, French, German, Italian, Spanish, Danish, or Dutch. In addition, all abstract supplements from the same period published in *Radiology, American Journal of Radiology, Journal of Vascular and Interventional Radiology, European Radiology*, and *Surgical Endoscopy* were searched manually. Relevant papers were also identified from the reference lists of the papers previously obtained through the search and from abstracts from recent international meetings. Further, the six major companies that produce commercial RF electrodes were contacted: *Valleylab*®, Boulder, CO. (formerly: Radionics®); *RITA*® Medical Systems, Mountain View, CA; *Boston Scientific*® (formerly: Radiotherapeutics®), Natick, MA; *Berchtold*®, Tuttlingen, Germany; *Invatec*®, Roncadelle, Italy; and *Celon AG Medical Instruments*®, Teltow, Germany.[2−7]

For each basic electrode design, a generic name has been defined which had to be unequivocal, descriptive of the electrode's main working principle and as concise as possible. In a second step, these basic names have been combined to describe the combination electrode designs. In a third step, a logical description of the combined use of more than one RF electrode in multiple electrode systems has been worked out.

3.   RESULTS

3.1.   Single-Shaft Electrodes Basic Designs (Table 1; Figs. 1–3)

3.1.1.   Plain Electrodes

The first experiments with RFA on liver tissue were performed with *plain* metal electrodes. The ablation diameter was very limited, due to a rapid rise in electric impedance with current shut-off. To overcome size limitations in RFA, modified single-shaft electrodes have been developed and tested since 1994. Four approaches have been followed: internal cooling (cooled electrodes), enlargement of the electric field and the electrode-tissue interface (expandable electrodes), saline perfusion through the electrode into the tissue (wet electrodes), and bipolar design (bipolar electrodes).[8,9]

Table 1. Single-shaft radiofrequency electrodes, basic designs: proposed terminology

Current proposal	IWGIGTA proposal	Other synonyms in literature
Plain	–	
Cooled	Internally cooled	Perfusion, closed perfusion, perfused, Internally cooled-tip
Single cooled	Single internally cooled	
Cluster cooled	Cluster internally cooled	Array, clustered internally cooled, triple cooled
Expandable		
Multitined	Multitined	Retractable, umbrella, Christmas tree, multiple hooked, array, anchor, multi-probe needle
Coiled	–	
Bipolar	–	
Wet	Perfusion	Liquid, virtual, saline, saline-enhanced, saline-augmented, saline infusion, perfused, open perfused, saline solution perfusion

Basic electrode designs

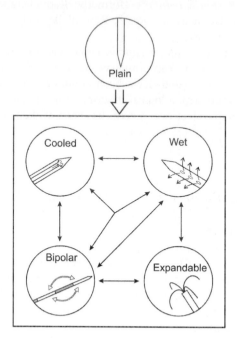

Figure 1. Five basic designs of RF ablation electrodes (plain, cooled, wet, expandable, and bipolar) have led to the development of six combination designs (cooled-wet, expandable-wet, bipolar-wet, bipolar-cooled, bipolar-expandable, and bipolar-cooled-wet).

Single shaft electrodes, combined designs

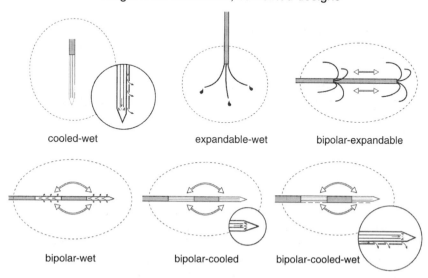

Figure 2. Single-shaft electrodes: basic designs.

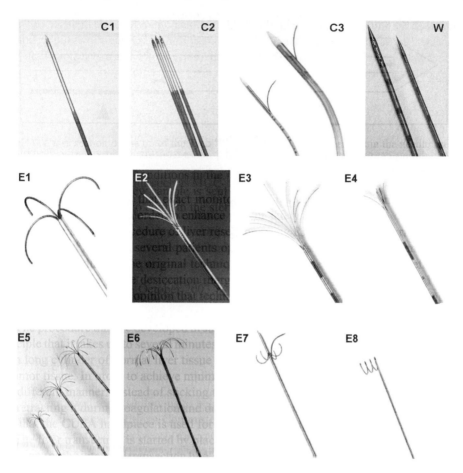

Figure 3. Examples of commercial electrodes with a basic design C(ooled) 1 = Radionics® Cool-tip RF® single 3-cm tip; C(ooled) 2 = Radionics® Cool-tip RF® luster; C(ooled) 3 = Convatec® MIRAS IOC® and Convatec® MIRAS LC® (top to bottom); W(et) = Berchtold® HiTT® 1-cm tip/1.2 mm diameter and 1.5-cm tip/2 mm diameter; E(xpandable) 1 = RITA® model 30; E(xpandable) 2 = RITA® model 70; E(xpandable) 3 = RITA® model 90/StarBurst XL®; E(xpandable) 4 = RITA® StarBurst SD; E(xpandable) 5 = Boston Scientific® LeVeen® 2-,3-, and 3.5 cm; E(xpandable) 6 = Boston Scientific® LeVeen® 4 cm; E(xpandable) 7 = Convatec® MIRAS LN®; E(xpandable) 8 = Convatec® MIRAS RC®.

3.1.2. Cooled Electrode

The *cooled* electrode[10–15] is a hollow electrode that contains an inner cannula, dividing the space inside the electrode into a concentric outer, and inner lumen. The inner lumen is used to deliver a chilled fluid to the tip of the electrode and the outer returns the fluid to an external collection unit. The fluid does not leave the electrode. This way, the tip is internally cooled to a temperature below 25 °C to prevent charring of the tissue immediately adjacent to the tip. In a *cluster cooled* electrode,[16] three parallel cooled electrodes have been mounted on the same shaft in a triangular fashion with an interelectrode distance of 5 mm. The electrodes are activated simultaneously. The larger contact surface allows higher current densities with less charring around the tip and therefore larger thermal lesions than with single cooled electrodes.[16]

3.1.3.   Expandable Electrodes

An expandable electrode is inserted as a straight insulated needle into the tissue. Once in the desired position, the active electrode is deployed from the hollow shaft of the probe. Two types exist: the *multitined* type and the *coiled* type.

Multitined electrodes[17] are an array of 4 to 12 curved electrode tines ("prongs") that are deployed from the hollow needle tip in an umbrella-like or Christmas tree-like fashion. The coagulation shape follows the configuration of the deployed prongs. The power is distributed over a wider surface area, therefore current density and the chance of charring decrease.

A *coiled* electrode has a spring that leaves the tip and that is deployed perpendicularly to the shaft.[18]

3.1.4.   Wet Electrode

The *wet* electrode[19,20] (Figs. 1–4) consists of a hollow electrode with one or more holes at the uninsulated distal end through which an isotonic or hypertonic saline solution is infused into the tissue. The infused saline improves thermal and electrical tissue conductivity, which allows for a greater than 10 fold increase in power deposition compared to a plain electrode.[21]

3.1.5.   Bipolar Electrodes

In *bipolar* electrodes, both electrodes are incorporated proximally and distally on the same neutral probe with a variable distance between them.[22,23] The electric current flows between the two electrodes, and no grounding pad is used.

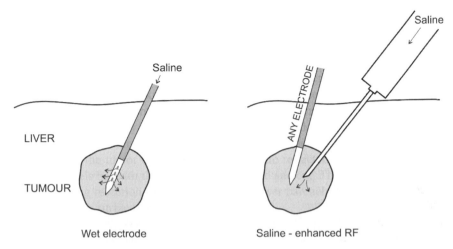

Figure 4. Wet electrode-RF ablation vs. saline-enhanced RF ablation

Table 2. Single-shaft radiofrequency electrodes, combination designs: proposed terminology

Current proposal	Synonyms in literature
Double combination designs	
Cooled-wet	Perfusion, perfused-cooled, wet-cooled, open perfused
Expandable-wet	Perfusion
Bipolar-wet	
Bipolar-cooled	
Bipolar-expandable	Bipolar
Bipolar-cooled-wet	
Triple combination designs	
Bipolar-cooled-wet	Bipolar perfused-cooled

3.2. Double Combination Electrode Designs (Table 2; Figs. 1, 5, and 6)

3.2.1. Cooled-Wet Electrode

The *cooled-wet* electrode allows continuous infusion of interstitial saline along the cooled electrode. The cooled-wet electrode yields larger ablation zones than both the wet and the cooled electrode separately.[24,25]

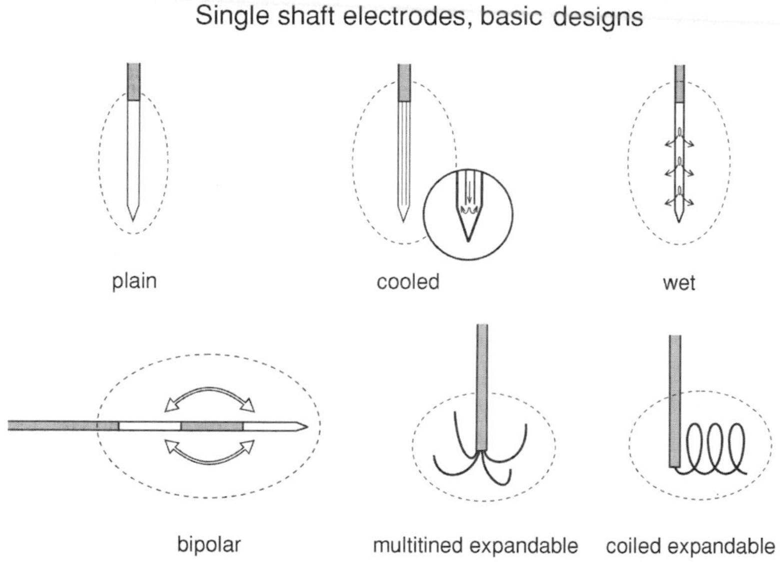

Figure 5. Single-shaft electrodes: combination designs

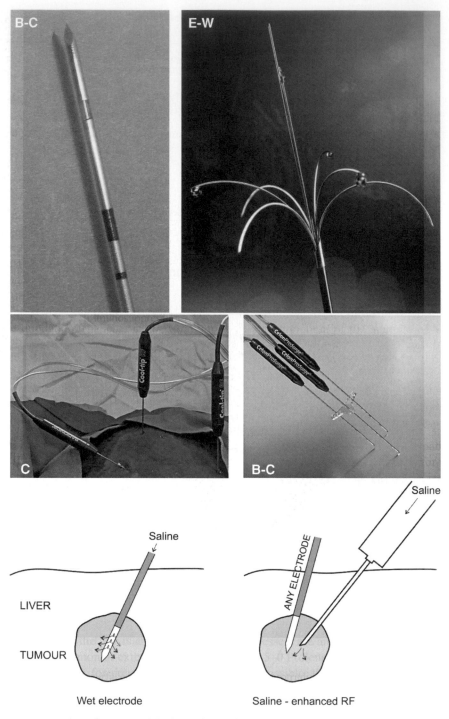

Figure 6. Examples of commercial electrodes with a combination design B(ipolar)-C(ooled) = CelonProSurge® 150T30 electrode; E(xpandable)-W(et) = RITA® model 100/StarBurst XLi® 70.

3.2.2.   Expandable-Wet

The *expandable-wet* electrode, which unites features of both techniques is more effective than the wet or expandable electrode separately in an experimental setting.[26,27]

3.2.3.   Bipolar-Wet Electrode

A *bipolar-wet* electrode consists of an insulated shaft with two electrodes, connected in a bipolar fashion and separated by an insulated portion. Saline flows into the tissue at both active parts.[28]

3.2.4.   Bipolar-Cooled Electrode

A *bipolar-cooled* electrode consists of an internally cooled and insulated shaft with two exposed electrode parts, connected in a bipolar fashion and separated by an insulated portion.[22]

3.2.5.   Bipolar-Expandable Electrode

A *bipolar-expandable* electrode consists of two expandable electrodes that are incorporated in parallel into one shaft.[29] Current flows between the two expanded parts.

3.3.   Triple Combination Electrode Designs (Table 2; Figs. 1 and 5)

3.3.1.   Bipolar-Cooled-Wet Electrode

A bipolar-cooled-wet electrode consists of a cooled-wet electrode with a second, more proximal exposed electrode part, connected in a bipolar fashion and separated by an insulated portion.[30]

3.4.   Multiple Electrode Systems (Table 3; Figs. 7 and 8)

Multiple electrode systems are defined as the combined use of more than one single-shaft electrode. Their use can be described according to the number of electrodes used, electric mode, activation mode, and location of the inserted electrodes. Multiple electrode systems have been built with many types of electrodes. The number of possible combinations using these different variables is infinite.

3.4.1.   Number of Electrodes Used

A multiple electrode system can consist of two (*dual*), three (*triple*), four (quadruple), or more electrodes.

Table 3. Multiple electrode systems: proposed terminology

Current proposal	Synonyms in literature
According to number	
Dual, triple, quadruple, etc.	
According to electric mode	
Monopolar	
Bipolar	
According to activation mode	
Consecutive	Sequential
Simultaneous	
Switching	Multipolar, sequential, alternative
According to site of insertion	
Unifocal	
Multifocal	
According to electrodes	
Plain electrode system	Multiprobe array, bipolar, Multibipolar, Multielectrode
Wet electrode system	Bipolar saline-enhanced
Cooled electrode system	
Expandable electrode system	
Cooled-wet electrode system	
Bipolar-cooled electrode system	Multipolar

3.4.2. Electric Mode

A multiple electrode system can be used in the *monopolar* mode.[29,31–35] The electric current flows from all the electrodes that have the same polarity toward the grounding pad. Alternatively, in the *bipolar* mode,[36–42] the current flows between two parallelly inserted electrodes or groups of electrodes. The inaccurate term "bipolar RFA" should be avoided, because it can cause confusion. Instead, authors should clearly describe whether they use a bipolar *single-shaft electrode* or whether they use the bipolar *mode* between two (or more) *parallelly* inserted electrodes *in multiple electrode systems*.

3.4.3. Activation Mode

Multiple electrodes can be activated *consecutively*[31,34,35]: the second electrode is activated after completion of the session of the first electrode etc. They can also be activated *simultaneously*,[29,32–34] or in a *switching* mode using a switch box.[29,34]

3.4.4. Insertion Site of the Electrodes

Usually, the multiple electrodes are inserted in the same part of the organ to treat the same tumor (*monofocal* RFA). Alternatively, two (or more) (groups of) electrodes can be inserted in a different part of the organ, to obtain a simultaneous treatment at different locations (*multifocal* RFA, e.g. *bifocal* or *trifocal* RFA).[43] For multifocal RFA, the interposition of

Multiple electrode systems

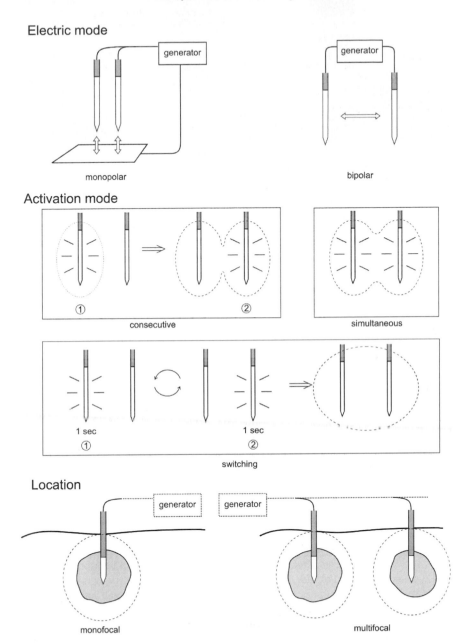

Figure 7. Multiple electrode systems: they can be characterized by the number of electrodes used (not shown), the electric mode (example with two plain electrodes), activation mode (example with two plain electrodes), site of insertion (example with one plain electrode at each location), and (not shown) type of single-shaft electrodes used.

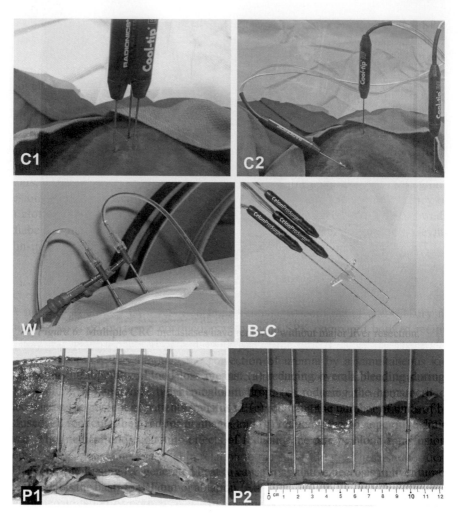

Figure 8. Examples of multiple electrode systems C(ooled) 1 = three Radionics® Cool-tip RF® single 3-cm tip with monofocal insertion in the switching and monopolar mode to treat three one large tumor C(ooled) 2 = three Radionics® Cool-tip RF® single 3-cm tip with multifocal insertion in the switching and monopolar mode to treat three different sites at the same time W(et) = two Berchtold® HiTT® electrodes with monofocal insertion in the bipolar mode to treat one large tumor B(ipolar)-C(ooled) = three CelonProSurge® 150T40 electrodes that will be used with monofocal insertion in the switching and bipolar mode to treat one large tumor P(lain) 1 = two rows (only one shown) of five plain metal electrodes of uneven lengths, spaced apart 2 cm and activated in a bipolar and simultaneous mode in ex vivo beef liver; note the triangular shape of the coagulation that closely matches the distribution of the unexposed parts of the electrodes P(lain) 2 = two rows (only one shown) of six plain metal electrodes of uneven lengths, spaced apart 2 cm and activated in a bipolar mode in ex vivo beef liver; the three pairs of electrodes left and the three pairs right have been activated consecutively; note the bilobar shape of the coagulation that closely matches the distribution of the unexposed parts of the electrodes.

Table 4. Wet electrode-RF ablation vs. saline-enhanced RF ablation

	Wet electrode RF ablation	Saline-enhanced RF ablation
Method of saline instillation	Saline infused through electrode	Saline injected through separate needle
Site of saline exit	Side-holes of electrode	Tip of separate needle
Device	Dedicated electrode	Saline injection can be combined with any electrode
Timing of saline instillation	Usually bolus pre-RF ablation plus continuous infusion during RF ablation	Usually bolus pre-RF ablation

a switch box between electrodes and generator is necessary. This switch box is usually programed to distribute the current in a switching mode to the different locations, but it can be programmed in any activation mode as well as in any electric mode [Mulier, unpublished data].

3.4.5. Types of Electrodes Used in Multiple Electrode Systems

Multiple electrode systems can be made with any of the available single-shaft electrodes. The following systems have been described in the literature.

A *plain electrode system* consists of two or more plain electrodes that are inserted in a parallel way into the tissue. Two electrodes can be arranged in a bipolar mode,[29,36] or current can be applied simultaneously to multiple electrodes in a monopolar mode.[29,31,32] A third option is to insert multiple plain electrodes in a parallel way, half of which are connected to the positive pole and half of which are connected to the negative pole.[37,38,42]

Similarly, by inserting two or more parallel electrodes of the same kind, a *wet electrode system*,[39,40,44] a *cooled electrode system*,[33,34] an *expandable electrode system*,[29,35,41,45] a *cooled-wet electrode system*[30,44] and a *bipolar-cooled electrode system*[7] have been described.

3.5. Saline-Enhanced RFA (Fig. 4, Table 4)

In *saline-enhanced RFA*,[46] saline is directly injected into the tissue near the electrode tip.[47-50] The injection needle is not incorporated into the electrode, in contrast to the wet electrode (Fig. 4; Table 4). Saline-enhanced RFA can be performed in combination with any of the existing electrodes and multiple electrode systems. Saline-enhancement has been reported for *cooled* electrodes,[47,49-51] *multiple plain* electrodes,[46] and *expandable* electrodes.[48] Saline is usually injected as a bolus prior to RFA,[47,49,50] in contrast to the wet electrode, with which usually a continuous infusion after a pre-RFA bolus is used. Reports on saline-enhanced RFA should specify details on the injection method.

4. DISCUSSION

Research and clinical application of soft tissue RFA is booming. Proposals have recently been launched to standardize reporting on RFA. A recent paper from the IWGIGTA (International Working Group on Image-Guided Tumor Ablation) proposes standardized terms for various aspects in the broad field of image-guided tumor destruction.[1] Other papers focused on standardized reporting of one specific aspect of RFA, such as RFA treatment protocols,[52] size and geometry of RFA lesions,[18] and severity of complications.[53,54] All these efforts at standardization are crucial to improve scientific communication on RFA.

The IWGIGTA proposal described most of the commercial electrodes that were available at that moment (Table 1). It did not yet cover the many new commercial and experimental electrodes, as well as several "multiple electrode systems" that have been introduced since. The aim of this article is to update and adapt the existing classification and to present a logical and easily adoptable terminology for the generic classification of all RF electrodes and multiple electrode systems.

At present, the naming of many new experimental and commercial electrode types is much influenced by *subjective factors*: personal preferences of the inventors or major users, or fancy names for marketing purposes. In order to obtain a logical terminology for RF electrodes that was scientific and acceptable to all, we first developed *objective criteria* that had to be fulfilled to name the basic electrode designs. These names had to be unequivocal, descriptive of the electrode's main working principle and as short as possible. A short name was crucial to be able to combine these names to describe the combination designs in a second step. As a logical consequence of these objective criteria, two of the terms for the basic designs of the IWGIGTA proposal had to be adapted:

In the present terminology proposal, the term *wet electrode* replaces "perfusion electrode." The term "perfusion electrode" is still equivocal: this name is currently being used in the literature for both the *wet electrode*, which is perfused with saline which leaves the tip through small holes ("open perfusion electrode,"[44] or "externally perfused electrode"[55]); and for the *cooled electrode*, which is perfused with water which does not leave the electrode ("closed perfusion electrode",[56] or "internally perfused electrode"[55]). Further, the IWGIGTA classification uses the same term "perfusion electrode" for both the *wet* and the *cooled-wet* electrode, which clearly have a different design and efficacy.[25,57]

The term we propose, *wet electrode*, is short, unequivocal, descriptive of the electrode's main working principle and used by several pioneering authors in this field.[21,58,59] It is currently being used as part of the name to describe several experimental electrodes and multiple electrode systems.[27,44,57,60]

The term "internally" cooled' electrode from the IWGIGTA classification has been shortened to *cooled* electrode, which is equally clear (as an externally cooled electrode does not exist) but shorter and easier to combine in names such as *cooled-wet; bipolar-cooled,* etc. The system of short unequivocal names for the basic electrode designs allows the easy introduction of combined names for electrodes with a *combination design*, even for future electrodes that have yet to be designed. Conversely, the clarity of the combined names facilitates the understanding of the design.

The introduction of the concept of *multiple electrode systems*, that consist of the combination of more than one single-shaft electrode and that can be used in many modes, was essential to cover this most recent and promising evolution in RFA technology. The names of these modes have been standardized too. The unequivocal term *switching* mode replaces the term "sequential," which has been used as a synonym for both the *switching* and the *consecutive* mode.

Due to superficial similarities, saline-enhanced RFA and wet electrode-mediated RFA are often confounded. It is hoped that the present definition, the table and the illustration can help to clearly distinguish these different technologies.

5.   ACKNOWLEDGMENT

The authors wish to thank Marie-Bernadette Jacqmain for the illustrations and Christian Deneffe for layout.

REFERENCES

1. Goldberg SN, Charboneau JW, Dodd GD III, Dupuy DE, Gervais DA, Gillams AR, Kane RA, Lee FT Jr, Livraghi T, McGahan JP, Rhim H, Silverman SG, Solbiati L, Vogl TJ, Wood BJ. Image-guided tumor ablation: proposal for standardization of terms and reporting criteria. *Radiology.* 2003;228:335–345.
2. http://www.radionics.com/default-ab.shtml, accessed February 4th, 2004
3. http://www.ritamedical.com/, accessed February 4th, 2004.
4. http://www.bostonscientific.com/, accessed February 4th, 2004.
5. http://www.berchtold.de/2/main2.htm, accessed February 4th, 2004.
6. http://www.invatec.it/1024/index1024.htm, accessed February 4th, 2004.
7. http://www.celon.com/htdocs/11ech/efset1.htm, accessed June 30th 2004-07-27.
8. Denys AL, De Baere T, Kuoch V, Dupas B, Chevallier P, Madoff DC, Schnyder P, Doenz F. Radio-frequency tissue ablation of the liver: in vivo and ex vivo experiments with four different systems. *Eur Radiol.* 2003;13:2346–2352.
9. Pereira PL, Trubenbach J, Schenk M, Subke J, Kroeber S, Schaefer I, Remy CT, Schmidt D, Brieger J, Claussen CD. Radiofrequency ablation: in vivo comparison of four commercially available devices in pig livers. *Radiology.* 2004;232:482–490.
10. De Baere T, Elias D, Ducreux M, Dromain C, Kuoch V, El Din MG, Sobotka A, Lasser P, Roche A. Percutaneous radiofrequency ablation of hepatic metastases. Preliminary experience. *Gastroenterol Clin Biol.* 1999;23:1128–1133.
11. Goldberg SN, Gazelle GS, Solbiati L, Rittman WJ, Mueller PR. Radiofrequency tissue ablation: increased lesion diameter with a perfusion electrode. *Acad Radiol.* 1996;3:636–644.
12. Lencioni R, Goletti O, Armillotta N, Paolicchi A, Moretti M, Cioni D, Donati F, Cicorelli A, Ricci S, Carrai M, Conte PF, Cavina E, Bartolozzi C. Radio-frequency thermal ablation of liver metastases with a cooled-tip electrode needle: results of a pilot clinical trial. *Eur Radiol.* 1998;8:1205–1211.
13. Lorentzen T. A cooled needle electrode for radiofrequency tissue ablation: thermodynamic aspects of improved performance compared with conventional needle design. *Acad Radiol.* 1996;3:556–563.
14. Solbiati L, Goldberg SN, Ierace T, Livraghi T, Meloni F, Dellanoce M, Sironi S, Gazelle GS. Hepatic metastases: percutaneous radio-frequency ablation with cooled-tip electrodes. *Radiology.* 1997;205:367–373.
15. Trübenbach J, Huppert PE, Pereira PL, Ruck P, Claussen CD. Radiofrequency ablation of the liver in vitro: increasing the efficacy by perfusion probes. *Rofo Fortschr Geb Rontgenstr Neuen Bildgeb Verfahr.* 1997;167:633–637.

16. Goldberg SN, Solbiati L, Hahn PF, Cosman E, Conrad JE, Fogle R, Gazelle GS. Large-volume tissue ablation with radio frequency by using a clustered, internally cooled electrode technique: laboratory and clinical experience in liver metastases. *Radiology.* 1998;209:371–379.

17. Le Veen RF, Fox RL, Schneider PD, Hinrichs S. Large volume porcine liver ablation with the use of a percutaneous expandable electrosurgical probe. *JVIR 7* 2003;(1, part 2):217–218.

18. Mulier S, Ni Y, Miao Y, Rosiere A, Khoury A, Marchal G, Michel L. Size and geometry of hepatic radiofrequency lesions. *Eur J Surg Oncol.* 2003;29:867–878.

19. Hoey MF, Mulier PM, Shake JG. Intramural ablation using radiofrequency energy via screw-tip catheter and saline electrode. *PACE.* 1995;18 (II):917.

20. Livraghi T, Goldberg SN, Monti F, Bizzini A, Lazzaroni S, Meloni F, Pellicano S, Solbiati L, Gazelle GS. Saline-enhanced radio-frequency tissue ablation in the treatment of liver metastases. *Radiology.* 1997;202:205–210.

21. Leveillee RJ, Hoey MF. Radiofrequency interstitial tissue ablation: wet electrode. *J Endourol.* 2003;17:563–577.

22. Mack M, Straub R, Desinger K, Balzer JO, Zangos S, Vogl TJ. MR guided interstitial bipolar RF thermometry (RFITT): in vitro evaluations and first clinical results. *Radiology.* 2000;217 (suppl):539.

23. Mack MG, Desinger K, Straub R, Stein T, Balzer JO, Vogl TJ. MR-guided bipolar RF-thermotherapy (RFITT): in vitro evaluations and first clinical results. *Eur Radiol.* 2002;12 (suppl 1):141.

24. Ni Y, Miao Y, Marchal G. Cooled-wet electrode. US patent no 6514251 B1, Feb 4, 2003. Priority date: August 14, 1998

25. Miao Y, Ni Y, Yu J, Marchal G. A comparative study on validation of a novel cooled-wet electrode for radiofrequency ablation. *Invest Radiol.* 2000;35:438–444.

26. Miao Y, Ni Y, Yu J, Marchal GJ. Optimization of radiofrequency ablation by using an 'expandable-wet' electrode: results of ex vivo experiment. *Radiology.* 1999;213:102.

27. Miao Y, Ni Y, Yu J, Zhang H, Baert A, Marchal G. An ex vivo study on radiofrequency tissue ablation: increased lesion size by using an "expandable-wet" electrode. *Eur Radiol.* 2001;11:1841–1847.

28. Mulier P, Hoey M. Method and apparatus for creating a bi-polar virtual electrode used for the ablation of tissue. US Patent no 6238393 B1, May 29, 2001. Priority date July 6, 1999.

29. Haemmerich D, Tungjitkusolmun S, Staelin ST, Lee FT Jr, Mahvi DM, Webster JG. Finite-element analysis of hepatic multiple probe radio-frequency ablation. *IEEE Trans Biomed Eng.* 2002;49:836–842.

30. Lee JM, Han JK, Kim SH, Lee JY, Kim DJ, Lee MW, Cho GG, Han CJ, Choi BI. Saline-enhanced hepatic radiofrequency ablation using a perfused-cooled electrode: comparison of dual probe bipolar mode with monopolar and single probe bipolar modes. *Korean J Radiol.* 2004;5:121–127.

31. Wright AS, Haemmerich DG, Chachati L, Webster JG, Mahvi DM, Lee FT. Hepatic radiofrequency ablation with multiple active electrodes is superior to conventional overlapping technique in an ex vivo model. *Radiology.* 2002;225 (suppl):639.

32. Goldberg SN, Gazelle GS, Dawson SL, Rittman WJ, Mueller PR, Rosenthal DI. Radiofrequency tissue ablation using multiprobe arrays: greater tissue destruction than multiple probes operating alone *Radiology.* 1994;193:S281.

33. Gillams AR, Lees WR. Optimisation of treatment strategy using cooled-tip radiofrequency electrodes in ex vivo liver. *European Radiol.* 2001;11(suppl A):171.

34. Lee JM, Rhim H, Han JK, Youn BJ, Kim SH, Choi BI. Dual-probe radiofrequency ablation: an in vitro experimental study in bovine liver. *Invest Radiol.* 2004;39:89–96.

35. Shirato K, Morimoto M, Tomita N, Kokawa A, Sugimori K, Saito T, Tanaka K. Hepatocellular carcinoma: percutaneous radiofrequency ablation using expandable needle electrodes and the double-insertion technique. *Hepatogastroenterology.* 2002;49:1481–1483.

36. Jones CD, McGahan JP, Gu W, Brock JM. Percutaneous liver ablation using bipolar radiofrequency electrocautery. *Radiology.* 1995;197:140.

37. Mulier S, Ni Y, Mulier P, Marchal G, Michel L. Multi-bipolar electrode system. Patent application GB0318661A0, August 8, 2003.

38. Mulier S, Ni Y, Mulier P, Marchal G, Michel L. Linear radiofrequency coagulation. Patent application GB0324458A0, October 21, 2003.

39. Burdio F, Guemes A, Burdio JM, Castiella T, De Gregorio MA, Lozano R, Livraghi T. Hepatic lesion ablation with bipolar saline-enhanced radiofrequency in the audible spectrum. *Academic Radiol.* 1999;6:680–686.

40. Burdio F, Guemes A, Burdio JM, Navarro A, Sousa R, Castiella T, Cruz I, Burzaco O, Lozano R. Bipolar saline-enhanced electrode for radiofrequency ablation: results of experimental study of in vivo porcine liver. *Radiology*. 2003;229:447–456.
41. Lee FT, Staelin ST, Haemmerich D, Tungjitkusolmun S, Johnson CD, Mahvi DM. Bipolar RF produces larger zones of necrosis than conventional monopolar RF in pig livers. *Radiology*. 2000;217(suppl):229.
42. Gananadha S, Morris DL. Novel in-line multielectrode radiofrequency ablation considerably reduces blood loss during liver resection in an animal model. *ANZ J Surg*. 2004;74:482–485.
43. Lee FT, Haemmerich D, Wright AW, Mahvi DM, Sampson LA, Webster JG. Multiple probe radiofrequency ablation: pilot study in an animal model. *JVIR* 2003;14:1437–1442.
44. Lee JM, Han JK, Kim SH, Sohn KL, Choi SH, Choi BI. Bipolar radiofrequency ablation in ex vivo bovine liver with the open-perfused system versus the cooled-wet system. *Eur J Radiol*. 2005 Jun;54(3):408–417.
45. Xu H, Xie X, Lu M, Chen J, Yin X, Xu Z, Liu G. Ultrasound-guided percutaneous thermal ablation of hepatocellular carcinoma using microwave and radiofrequency ablation. *Clin Radiol*. 2004;59:53–61.
46. Solbiati L, Ierace T, Goldberg SN, Sironi S, Livraghi T, Fiocca R, Servadio G, Rizzatto G, Mueller PR, Del Maschio A, Gazelle GS. Percutaneous US guided radiofrequency tissue ablation of liver metastases: treatment and follow up in 16 patients. *Radiology*. 1997;202:195–203.
47. Lobo SM, Afzal KS, Ahmed M, Kruskal JB, Lenkinski RE, Goldberg SN. Radiofrequency ablation: modeling the enhanced temperature response to adjuvant NaCl pretreatment. *Radiology*. 2004;230:175–182.
48. Lubienski A, Wirth-Jaworski L, Hahn T, Bitsch R, Lubienski K, Dechow C, Kauffmann G, Düx M. Tissue modulation during radiofrequency ablation in an experimental liver perfusion model. *Eur Radiol*. 2003;13(suppl 2):S114
49. Kim YK, Lee JM, Kim SW, Kim CS. Combined radiofrequency ablation and hot saline injection in rabbit liver. *Invest Radiol*. 2003;38:725–732.
50. Lee JM, Kim YK, Lee YH, Kim SW, Li CA, Kim CS. Percutaneous radiofrequency thermal ablation with hypertonic saline injection: in vivo study in a rabbit liver model. *Korean J Radiol*. 2003;4:27–34.
51. Solbiati L, Goldberg SN, Livraghi T, Meloni F, Ierace T, Cova L. Radiofrequency thermal ablation: increased treatment effect with saline pre-treatment. *Radiology*. 2000;217(suppl):607.
52. Helton WS. Minimizing complications with radiofrequency ablation for liver cancer: the importance of properly controlled clinical trials and standardized reporting. *Ann Surg*. 2004;239:459–463.
53. Buscarini E, Buscarini L. Radiofrequency thermal ablation with expandable needle of focal liver malignancies: complication report. *Eur Radiol*. 2004;14:31–37.
54. Omary RA, Bettmann MA, Cardella JF, Bakal CW, Schwartzberg MS, Sacks D, Rholl KS, Meranze SG, Lewis CA; Society of Interventional Radiology Standards of Practice Committee. Quality improvement guidelines for the reporting and archiving of interventional radiology procedures. *J Vasc Interv Radiol*. 2003;14(9 Pt 2):S293–S295.
55. Kettenbach J, Blum M, Kilanowicz E, Schwaighofer SM, Lammer J. Percutaneous radiofrequence-ablation of liver cell carcinoma: a current overview. *Radiologe*. 2004;44:330–338.
56. Schmidt D, Trubenbach J, Konig CW, Brieger J, Duda S, Claussen CD, Pereira PL. Radiofrequenzablation ex vivo: Vergleich der Effektivität von impedance control mode versus manual control mode unter Verwendung einer geschlossen perfundierten Cluster-Ablationssonde. *Rofo Fortschr Geb Rontgenstr Neuen Bildgeb Verfahr*. 2003;175:967–972.
57. Ni Y, Miao Y, Mulier S, Yu J, Baert AL, Marchal G. A novel 'cooled-wet' electrode for radiofrequency ablation. *Eur Radiol*. 2000;10:852–854.
58. Miao Y, Ni Y, Mulier S, Yu J, De Wever I, Penninckx F, Baert AL, Marchal G. Treatment of VX2 liver tumor in rabbits with "wet" electrode mediated radio-frequency ablation. *Eur Radiol*. 2000;10:188–194.
59. Hänsler J, Witte A, Strobel D, Wein A, Bernatik T, Pavel M, Muller W, Hahn EG, Becker D. Radio-Frequency-Ablation (RFA) with wet electrodes in the treatment of primary and secondary liver tumours. *Ultraschall Med*. 2003;24:27–33.
60. Gangi A, Guth S, Imbert J. Interest of radiofrequency liver tissue ablation with a bipolar-wet electrode. *Eur Radiol*. 2003;13(suppl 1):477.

Minimal Blood Loss Radio Frequency Assisted Liver Resection Technique

MIROSLAV MILICEVIC and PREDRAG BULAJIC
The First Surgical Clinic, Institute for Digestive Diseases, University Clinical Center of Belgrade, Belgrade, Serbia and Montenegro

1.   INTRODUCTION

Liver surgery developed rapidly during the past 50 years, when practically all major abdominal operations were already routine practice in surgical departments worldwide. Better understanding of liver anatomy, physiology, and hepatic cell biology coupled with intraoperative ultrasound facilitated the performance of anatomical liver resections and resulted in the development of many surgical techniques. The mortality and morbidity associated with major liver resection significantly decreased in HPB centers of excellence and patients were offered safe and efficient surgery.

Nevertheless, liver surgery still remains a complex surgical procedure in general surgical units, especially in developing countries, where experienced and skilled surgeons as well as significant resources are not available. Intraoperative blood loss is a major concern for surgeons operating on the liver since it is associated with a significantly higher rate of postoperative complications and shorter long-term survival.[1]

Many different surgical techniques evolved during the past half-century in an attempt to reduce intraoperative blood loss during division of liver parenchyma and facilitate safer liver resections. Intraoperative blood loss can be decreased by performing operations in hypotensive anesthesia and by using vascular inflow and outflow control. All these procedures have their indications, hemodynamic consequences, and limitations mainly in patients with chronic liver disease and when doing nonanatomical resections.

Division of liver parenchyma can be done by simple procedures like cutting with a scalpel or crushing the tissue with fingers or clamps or using sophisticated forms of mechanical energy like ultrasonic dissectors, harmonic scalpel, compressive bipolar diathermy, floating ball devices, and hydroscissors. All these procedures are less efficient in cirrhotic livers and when doing nonanatomical resections.[2-5] A notable advance in liver surgery has been the increased use of parenchymal sparing, segmental resections, which has contributed to the improved perioperative results.

A new technique using radio frequency (RF) energy to coagulate liver resection margins and perform tissue sparing, practically bloodless liver resection is described.

N. A. Habib and R. Canelo (eds.), Liver and Pancreatic Diseases Management, 75–88.
© *2006 Springer. Printed in The Netherlands.*

2.   THE TECHNIQUE

All patients included into this study met the following criteria: (a) no extrahepatic spread of the disease, (b) respectability of the lesion or lesions with adequate margins, (c) no obstructive jaundice, (d) adequate remnant liver, and (e) no simultaneous operative procedures on other organs. Preoperative work-up of the patients is along the usual clinical guidelines. Special emphasis is placed on accurate preoperative tumor imaging by CT or NMR and planning the extent of resection. The lidocaine test to assess hepatic reserve is done in all patients with large or multiple liver tumors. No preoperative tumor biopsies are done. If the patient is to be operated for CRC metastases, a thorough preoperative search for local recurrence and disseminated disease is conducted. Tumor markers are studied in all potential candidates with malignant disease. If intraperitoneal seeding is suspected, prior to the abdominal incision, a diagnostic and staging laparoscopy is done.

Under general anesthesia a midline incision with a right sagittal prolongation (J incision) without opening the diaphragm was used in all patients. Intra-abdominal adhesions and the falciform ligament are divided. The peritoneal cavity is thoroughly examined for evidence of extrahepatic spread and local recurrence. A Thompson retractor is placed and positioned to ensure good exposure of the liver. The tumor-containing liver lobe is mobilized in a standard way to the extent necessary for the intended resection, avoiding unnecessary liver mobilization and manipulation.

Intraoperative ultrasound assisted by bimanual palpation is routinely done to determine the accurate position, extent, and number of the tumors. Determining the precise relation of the tumor mass to the hepatic veins and glissonian pedicles is crucial. The upper and lower surface of the liver is marked with diathermy in order to provide a road map for the resection. It is important to clearly mark the path of the resection line, since after RF is used the parenchyma becomes desiccated and hardened rendering further palpation and intraoperative ultrasound useless in determining the tumor edge. In the RF resection technique, we developed and employ it is essential to mark the undersurface of the liver as well. If seeding is present a biopsy is done.

The standard surgical technique that includes hepatic inflow occlusion (Pringle's maneuver) and extrahepatic or intrahepatic control of the hepatic veins was not performed. Low central venous pressure and the Trendelenburg position (patient in 15° head down position) were not used during liver parenchymal transection.

Coagulative desiccation is produced using the 1 or 3 cm water cooled-tip single RF probe (needle in the text) and a 500-kHz Generator (Radionics Europe, Model RFG-3D, N.V., Wettdren, Belgium). The generator is capable of producing 100 W of power (single electrode) and allows measurements of the generator output, tissue impedance, and electrode tip temperature. The needle contains a 1 or 3 cm exposed electrode, a thermocouple on the tip to monitor temperature and impedance, and three coaxial cannulae through which chilled (4–10 °C) sterile distilled water is forced by a rotary pump during RF energy application (Fig. 1). We use chilled distilled water instead of saline. Cooling of the tip prevents tissue boiling and cavitations immediately adjacent to the electrode.

The RS232 port of the Radionics generator is connected to a notebook computer running a specially designed software for the authors that monitors RF emission time (min), total delivered current (Coulombs), and maximal delivered current (mA). Since the RF generator was used for coagulating normal liver tissue, instead of tumor tissue for which it was

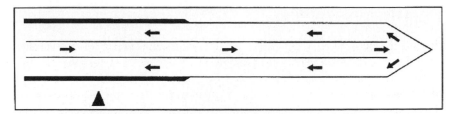

Figure 1. Cross section of the tip of the Tyco "cool-tip" needle. The channels in the needle used for cooling the tip with chilled distilled water are shown (pressure generated by the pump).

designed, the authors felt that exact monitoring of relevant output parameters and their registration was needed in order to enhance patient safety.

The principle and procedure of liver resection using RF energy was described in detail by Weber et al.[6] The first several patients operated in our series (during December 2001) were done according to the original technique. We found the technique to be effective in creating coagulative tissue desiccation margins that are safe to cut with a surgical scalpel with no blood loss. In our opinion that technique, although very effective, took a long time and created desiccated margins that were unnecessarily large.

The procedure that we developed in January–February 2002 is based on the same Habib principle that it takes up to several minutes to coagulate and desiccate a centimeter wide and 3 cm long cylinder of normal liver tissue instead of the 20 min it takes for the same effect in tumor tissue. In order to achieve minimal safe desiccated margins, we use the electrode in a different manner. Instead of sticking the electrode through the entire liver parenchyma and retracting it during coagulation and desiccation, we prefer to use the needle in a similar way that the CUSA handpiece is used for advancing through liver parenchyma.

The liver transection is started by placing the needle onto the liver surface marked with diathermy as the intended transection line. The active part of the needle (1 or 3 mm depending on the needle used) is brought into contact with the liver surface horizontally (along the long axis). This causes superficial desiccation of the liver surface (pale tissue, 2–4 mm wide) along the marked transection line. The needle is then inserted into the liver parenchyma parallel to the liver surface, 2–5 mm beneath the liver capsule, along the marked lines. RF energy is applied by rapidly increasing the output to maximum power, which, with the 3 mm tip needle, produces a smaller, ~30 mm long and 6 mm wide cylinder of desiccation in less than 10 s. Coagulative desiccation progresses upward to the liver surface causing the tissue to change to a pale color and boiling and bubbling of the tissue stops. After the cylinder of desiccated liver tissue is achieved, with the needle still in place, the desiccated tissue is cut with a surgical scalpel all the way to the nude tip of the needle (Fig. 2). The needle does not loose contact with tissue and the instrument does not switch off. The needle is advanced forward or backward in the same plane and the procedure is repeated. It is not necessary to monitor the generator parameters to determine when it is time to cut, although the computer will provide an audible signal if the current drops to below 0.3 mA. Using this technique a superficial hepatotomy on the anterior and posterior liver surface is performed outlining the desired transection plane. The resection advances from the surface into the depth of the liver and from the anterior to the posterior aspect of the liver. This is what we call a "sequential-coagulate–cut technique". Multiple rapid coagulate–cut cycles are needed

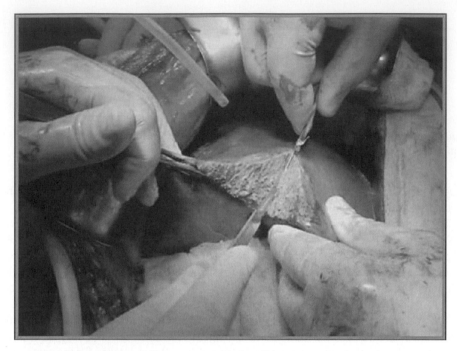

Figure 2. The "sequential-coagulate–cut technique" The needle is advanced, coagulated liver parenchyma is cut with a surgical scalpel all the way to the needle tip. The liver is transected without bleeding.

to achieve transection of the full thickness of the liver parenchyma. As transection of liver parenchyma progresses small tributaries (>3 mm) to the glissonian sheets and hepatic veins are identified, isolated, desiccated, and cut by scalpel. Desiccation of large glissonian sheets and tributaries to the hepatic veins is possible, but it is time consuming (heath sink effect) and application of unnecessary RF energy is needed. We prefer to dissect, clamp, cut, and tie these structures. Major hepatectomies, segmentectomies, and wedge resections were performed using this technique in our series (Fig. 3).

The same "sequential-coagulate–cut technique" is used when performing extra-anatomical resections for tumors located at the dome of the liver or inside liver parenchyma. The operation begins by marking the area on the liver surface approximately 1 cm away from the projection of the largest diameter of the tumor. A circular, convex plane of tissue transection through healthy liver parenchyma is developed by gradual spiral desiccation and cutting sequences along the marked circular line on the liver surface. When sufficient depth is reached, the tumor and liver parenchyma are retracted to one side and at a safe distance the vessels beneath the tumor are desiccated and cut. This ensures minimal blood loss, tissue sparing resection of tumors within the liver parenchyma which are sometimes not visible from the surface (Fig. 4a,b).

The "sequential-coagulate–cut technique" is done by two surgeons. One of the surgeons guides and directs the needle while the other surgeon cuts along the path of the needle. With

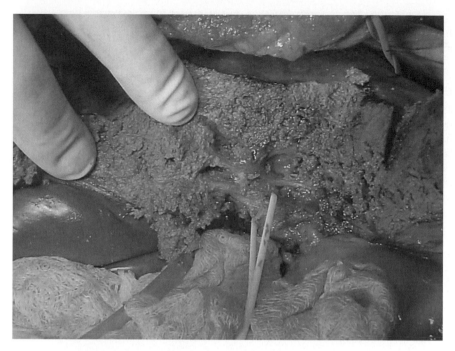

Figure 3. Glissonian sheets exposed during transection are not desiccated or coagulated.

experience, this process is fast, since the surgeon cutting at the site or adjacent to the needle can determine when adequate dissection and coagulation has been achieved. Extent of coagulation and desiccation depends on the energy, exposure time, and contact surface of the needle as well as the vicinity of large blood vessels (the "heat sink" effect). The cut surface is constantly sprayed with a controlled volume of sterile saline to facilitate conductivity.

Structures within the liver parenchyma are easily recognized as transection progresses. Glissonian sheets and veins can be coagulated or tied, depending on their diameter and the preference of the surgeon. Coagulation can be done from inside the resection margins to stop any residual or potential point of bleeding. Working with the electrode close to important structures is not a problem, providing direct contact and prolonged exposure are avoided. The Pringle maneuver was not applied in our series. A drain is placed at the site of the resection. The abdomen is subsequently closed in layers.

In all patients, biochemical liver function tests were monitored before and after resection within the first 24 h.

3.   PATIENTS AND RESULTS

Liver resection was done for different indications (Table 1). During a period ranging from December 1, 2001 to April 1, 2004 a total of 77 patients underwent 82 operations. The youngest patient was 18 years old and the oldest 78 years old (mode 60 years). Consecutive patients where liver only resection was done are included in the present series.

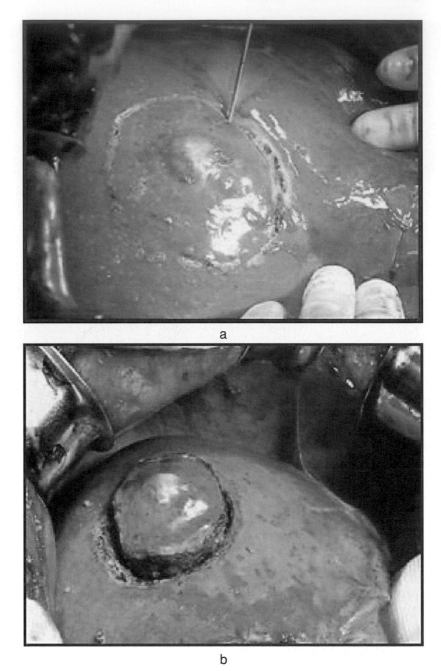

a

b

Figure 4. (a) The liver surface is marked around a metastases protruding at the dome of the liver and the transection line is developed. (b) The cone of tissue is resected by a spiral "sequential-coagulate–cut technique".

Table 1. Operated patients.

Indications for resection	No. of patients	% of patients
CRC metastases	54	65.9
Primary liver cancer	15	18.4
Giant liver hemangioma	3	3.7
Lung cancer metastases	2	2.4
Ovary cancer metastases	1	1.2
Gallbladder cancer	1	1.2
Liver hydatid cyst	1	1.2
Liver cystadenoma	1	1.2
Recurrent liver abscess	1	1.2
Liver actinomycosis	1	1.2
Solitary necrotic liver nodule	1	1.2
Metastasis—undetectable primary tumor	1	1.2
Total	82	100.0

Formal liver resection was done in 15 (18.3%) patients, right hepatectomy in 10 (12.2%) patients, left hepatectomy in 3 (3.7%) patients, extended left hepatectomy in 2 (2.4%) patients, segmentectomy in 40 (48.8%) patients, and extra-anatomical resection in 27 (32.9%) patients. Fifteen (18.3%) patients underwent segmental resection with concomitant extra-anatomical resection. Repeat liver resection for recurrent colorectal liver metastases was done in five (6.1%) patients. Seventeen (20.7%) patients underwent resection of both sides of the liver (Table 2).

The median time necessary for transection of the liver parenchyma was 82 min (mode 60 min). A total of 14 (17.0%) patients received blood transfusion (mean transfused blood volume 397 ml; mode 310 ml).

There was a transient increase in transaminase levels in 46 (56.1%) patients. There were 12 different postoperative complications. The most frequent complications were chest

Table 2. Type of liver resection.

Type of liver resection	No. of patients	% of patients
Minor resection		
Extra-anatomical	27	32.9
Segmentectomy	16	26.9
Two segments	20	17.0
Three segments	4	4.9
Major resection		
Right hepatectomy	10	12.2
Left hepatectomy	3	3.7
Extended left hepatectomy	2	2.4
Total	82	100.0

Table 3. Morbidity and mortality.

Type of complication	No. of patients
Pleural effusion	7
Perihepatic abscess[a]	4
Pneumonia	2
Wound infection	2
Pleural empyema	1
Postoperative liver failure[b]	1
Wound dehiscence[a]	1
Fracture of coli femoris	1
Stroke	1
Cerebral infarction[b]	1
Oliguria	1
Pseudomembraneous colitis[b]	1
Total	17[c]

[a] Reoperated.
[b] Died.
[c] Number of patients with complications (4 patients had more than 1 complication).

complications (10 patients). There were no biliary fistulas in the current series. The perioperative morbidity was 20.7% (17 patients) and four patients developed more than one complication. There was no intraoperative death. The mortality rate was 3.7%. The morbidity and mortality is presented in Table 3.

One patient was reoperated for sequestrated desiccated liver tissue and one other patient for abdominal wound dehiscence.

A 78-year-old patient died after liver resection for CRC liver metastases. In the early postoperative period, he developed oliguria that progressed to a short period of anuria with stable liver function. The kidney dysfunction was corrected but he soon developed uncontrollable diarrhea and sepsis in spite of intensive therapy. He died on the 28th day after operation. Autopsy revealed small sclerotic kidneys and pseudomembraneous colitis. Liver function was not affected by the operation.

A 75-year-old patient, operated for CRC metastases, died of cerebral infarction as verified by autopsy.

A 67-year-old patient operated for hepatocellular carcinoma died of intractable liver failure. She had a right hepatectomy done for a 5 cm lesion infiltrating the right main pedicle. The operation was uneventful, there was no blood loss. Liver function deteriorated in the postoperative period and the ensuing hepatic insufficiency was intractable.

There was no substantial blood loss related to the transection of the liver parenchyma. A total of 14 (17%) patients received blood transfusion. Detailed analysis reveals that 10 patients received less than 310 ml of blood (mean 277 ml, mode 310 ml) and the transfusion was not indicated by the operating surgeon but rather by the anesthetist who did not have a detailed knowledge of the RF resection procedure. Only four patients had acceptable indications for blood transfusion and received more than 2 U each (mean 700 ml). Blood loss in these patients was not related to the procedure on the liver but to difficult adhesiolysis and liver mobilization. The last 15 patients in the series did not receive blood transfusion.

4.   DISCUSSION

There are many different techniques for liver resection. Control of bleeding during liver resection is easiest when doing anatomical resections with demarcated boundaries between liver segments. Achieving demarcation of segments is not always simple for all of the segments and demands a good knowledge of liver anatomy and experience in hepatic surgery. The extent of resection is determined by the site, size, and spread of the tumor within the liver. This raises the question whether it is always necessary to utilize anatomical boundaries especially when resecting small, multiple, or bilateral tumors within the liver. When operating on cirrhotic livers and dealing with CRC metastases that are likely to recur, or when re-resecting an already resected liver, oncologically safe, tissue sparing procedures are preferred (Figs. 5 and 6).

During atypical liver resection intraoperative blood loss can further be reduced by applying the Pringle maneuver or vascular exclusion techniques. Interfering with liver blood supply is a time limited procedure that puts additional strain on hepatocytes.

RF assisted liver resection enables the surgeon to do atypical and typical liver resection without the need for Pringle's maneuver or vascular exclusion. When performing typical liver resection the electrode is guided along the demarcation line.

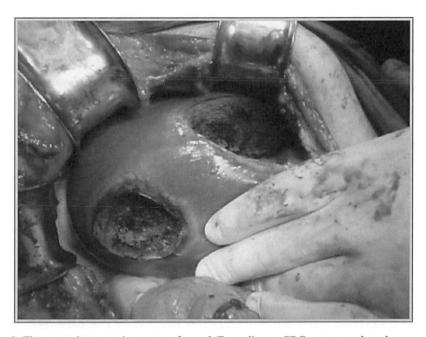

Figure 5. Tissue sparing resection was performed. Two adjacent CRC metastases have been removed without anatomical resection that would have demanded a hepatectomy.

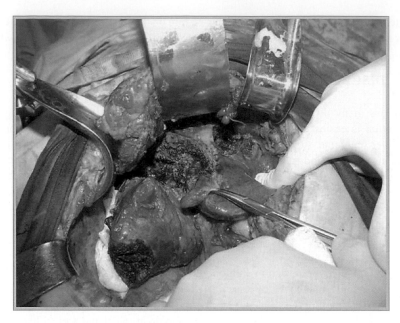

Figure 6. Multiple CRC metastases have removed without major liver resection.

Reducing intraoperative blood loss means: (a) reducing overall bleeding during tissue transection, (b) reducing the hemoglobin drop, (c) reducing the hematocrit drop, (d) decreasing the percent of patients transfused, (e) reducing the number of units of blood transfused, (f) reducing the need for drainage, and (g) reducing the postoperative drainage volume. The medical and economic effects of reducing the rate of blood transfusion are evident.

The concept of using RF generated heat to cause coagulative necrosis in liver tumors is not new and it is the basis for RF tumor ablation.[7-11] The innovative step with this technique is that the coagulation of normal liver parenchyma is very fast and elevated temperature causes desiccation and collagen bonding resulting in a type of "weld" at the resection line. Since all small vascular and biliary branches are "welded", the tissue is uniformly desiccated; postoperative bleeding and bile fistula are not probable.

The physics of RF are well defined. Body tissues are permeated by a saline solution and are relatively poor conductors. When RF current flows through the body it results in lost energy in the form of moving ions and water molecules. This "ionic agitation" causes friction and results in tissue heating that is directly proportional to current density (current flow per unit area of the electrode). This is different from direct heating by RF (standard diathermy). When using a standard diathermy heating is localized to the active electrode, as current density falls rapidly with distance from the electrode. Generated heat spreads into surrounding tissue by conduction until a steady state (thermal equilibrium) is achieved. The active electrode (high current densities), which is much smaller than the ground plate, heats tissue very rapidly resulting in rapid desiccation immediately surrounding the needle. This desiccated cellular debris functions as an insulator, reducing the size of the active electrode increasing the current density. Boiling, charring, tissue adherence, and associated thrombus formation results in dielectric breakdown if power is not terminated. This process is self-limiting as is the use of standard diathermy for transecting liver parenchyma. Obviously, the goal is to regulate current deposition to achieve maximum current density without overheating.[12]

Resistive heating produced by the RF generator used for transecting liver parenchyma in this study causes tissue desiccation and heat-based cellular death by inducing thermal coagulation necrosis. Irreversible cellular injury occurs when cells are heated to 46 °C for 60 min and occurs more rapidly as temperature rises. Immediate cellular damage and death results from protein coagulation of cytosolic and mitochondrial enzymes and nucleic acid–histone protein complexes.[13] Whether "coagulative necrosis" describes this thermal damage to normal liver tissue according to histopathological cell death criteria needs to be clarified.[12] The tissue is desiccated and difficult to stain for light microscopy. In order to perform RF assisted liver resection the optimal temperature range is probably between 65 and 100 °C. Heating over 100 °C results in tissue vaporization and charring and impedes the flow of current and restricts total energy deposition. Rapid overheating the tissue surrounding the active electrode leads to tissue charring, desiccation, sharp rise in impedance, and interrupts the RF circuit producing an effect similar to conventional monopolar diathermy units. Internally cooled electrodes, like the ones used in this study, allow greater RF energy deposition and rapid creation of desiccated liver tissue that can be safely cut without bleeding. Pulsing of energy has been used with RF generators to increase the mean intensity of energy deposition.

In developing the "sequential-coagulate–cut technique" the authors have noticed that the process is accelerated by spraying the area of the electrode with cold saline solution at regular intervals. The mechanisms responsible for the increase in the speed and extent of coagulation are multiple and not well understood. One hypothesis is that the high concentration of NaCl ions could increase the extent of coagulation necrosis by effectively increasing the area of the active electrode. Another hypothesis is that the effects of tissue vaporization are reduced (needle is in tissue contact despite formation of electrically insulating gases) or simply there is improved thermal conduction by diffusion of boiling solution into the tissues.[12] NaCl solution increases tissue conductivity enabling greater energy deposition, but on the other hand, with better conductivity greater energy is needed to heat tissues. It is the authors' practice, in the latter part of the series, to attach a baby infusion cannula with a drop counter adjacent to the insulated part of the internally cooled needle and to connect it to a sterile cooled NaCl infusion bag, so that during the entire process of liver parenchymal transection chilled saline drips (20–50 ml/min) onto the active part of the needle. The resection margins should be kept relatively dry during the transection procedure in order to achieve maximum efficacy.

RF assisted liver resection causes tissue desiccation and seals tissue by causing collagen, blood vessels, and smooth muscle to shrink. Liver tissue, small blood vessels, and bile ducts are first sealed and then cut by surgical scalpel, so the "sequential-coagulate–cut technique" is "clean" and the resulting cut surface is dry. Liver transection proceeds in a clean, practically bloodless, field where all structures can be identified before they are damaged. This permits accurate tissue removal and tissue sparing procedures. Since tissue temperatures are below 100 °C, there is no tissue burning and charring, no tissue boiling, no smoke or vapor, no tissue sticking, and no eschar formation. A minimal amount of foreign material (ties, sutures, clips, etc.) is left behind. Tissue sealing is permanent. No rebleeding and bile fistulas occur in the postoperative period.

There is concern about the inadvertent placement of the active electrode close to the liver hilum (contralateral thermal damage), the vena cava and intrahepatic portal pedicles of segments that are not to be resected. This could happen when placing the electrodes without accurate intraoperative U.S. guidance and in patients with distorted anatomy when utilizing the original Habib technique, especially if prolonged energy is applied. When using the "sequential-coagulate–cut technique" developed by the authors of this chapter, such an instance is not probable. The needle is always placed under direct visual guidance and short contact even with vital intrahepatic structures causes no damage. In an experimental study of cellular and vascular reactions in the liver to RF ablation with the wet needle applicators, it was demonstrated that large vessels (more than 10 mm) did not show any substantial changes after exposure to RF energy (included in the ablation zone). Therefore, tumors in close proximity to large blood vessels can be treated by RF tumor ablation with the wet electrode. The large perfusion volume in large vessels seems to be protective (cooling effect). Direct contact of the electrode and large vessels can lead to vessel wall damage and thrombus formation providing sufficient energy RF energy is applied long enough. Venous vessels less than 1 mm are completely thermally denaturated and destroyed. This effect on small vessels and bile ducts is important for RF assisted liver resection.[14]

The main advantage of RF assisted liver resection is that it makes atypical resection simple and bloodless. It is possible to do tissue sparing, oncologically correct, operations without inflow occlusion of the liver even at multiple sites in the liver. Unfortunately, it is difficult to classify these procedures as to what part of a segment or segments is resected, but since the tumor does not understand segmental anatomy, it might really be of no great importance if tumor-free margins are obtained. The "sequential-coagulate–cut technique" has several advantages: (a) it is under direct vision that the RF energy is applied and vital structures can be avoided, (b) vital structures can be ligated in order to save time and keep RF emission time (delivered energy) as short as possible, (c) resection can be extended to include devitalized liver parenchyma, (d) the margin of desiccated parenchyma left on the resected liver surface is minimal (several millimeters), (e) identification of pedicles and temporary clamping is possible, (f) it is possible to use this procedure on cirrhotic livers, and (g) if the tip of the electrode is carefully manipulated working around the VCI and portal vein is not a threat.

New, more powerful RF generators with advanced microprocessor control have been announced by some companies for tumor ablation. Nevertheless, when performing RF assisted liver resection the total amount of energy delivered needs to be as low as possible and constantly monitored. The benefit of using higher energy levels needs to be investigated.

The shape, type, ergonomics, elasticity, and concept of the RF energy handpiece for use in liver transection techniques is under study and development by several companies. Different concepts and designs of the RF applicator (wet, wet cooled, bipolar, bipolar wet, single, or multiple, etc.) have been produced and tested, but mostly for ablation purposes. Several companies (TissueLink, MCission) have designed disposable handpieces that can be used with standard RF generators (electrosurgical units) available at surgical departments. The Habib Sealer (MCission) is such a device. It is an economic, four-needle (paired two and two), bipolar handpiece that can connect to any electrosurgical unit. The Habib Sealer develops a coagulated zone of liver tissue only between the needles (electrodes) that can be cut by surgical scalpel.

The impact of RF assisted minimal blood loss liver resection techniques on how we do liver surgery remains to be evaluated. Any technique that is safe for the patient and effectively controls blood loss during liver transection even in nonanatomical resections and also provides oncologically safe resection margins needs further intense assessment.

5.   CONCLUSION

Developing RF assisted liver resection has affected the way we do liver resection. More difficult patients with more extensive disease are rendered operable. Vascular occlusion techniques are not used in routine practice anymore. Blood loss in RF assisted liver resection is minimal and disease-free margins can be obtained even with tissue sparing liver surgery. Altogether less extensive liver resections are performed because it is possible to control intraoperative bleeding more efficiently even in complex, atypical liver resections. Reoperation for liver recurrence is more often possible due to the initial tissue sparing procedure and the RF assisted safe technique for atypical liver resection. Biliary postoperative fistulae are infrequent. Operating time has been reduced. New RF application devices are being developed and tested. Liver resection has become simpler.

Further controlled studies are needed to evaluate the true value of RF assisted liver resection.

REFERENCES

1. Jarnagin W, Gonen M, Fong Y, DeMatteo R, Ben-Porat L, Little S, Corvera C, Weber S, Blumgart L. Improvement in perioperative outcome after hepatic resection. Analysis of 1,803 consecutive cases over the past decade. *Ann Surg.* 2002;4:397–407.
2. Tranberg KG, Rigotti P, Brackett KA, Bjornson HS, Fischer JE, Joffe SN. Liver resection. A comparison using the Nd-YAG laser, an ultrasonic surgical aspirator, or blunt dissection. *Am J Surg.* 1986;151:368–373.
3. Hansen PD, Isla AM, Habib NA. Liver resection using total vascular exclusion, scalpel division of the parenchyma, and a simple compression technique for hemostasis and biliary control. *J Gastrointest Surg.* 1999;3:537–542.
4. Yamamoto Y, Ikai I, Kume M, Sakai Y, Yamauchi A, Shinohara H, Morimoto T, Shimahara Y, Yamamoto M, Yamaoka Y. New simple technique for hepatic parenchymal resection using a Cavitron Ultrasonic Surgical Aspirator and bipolar cautery equipped with a channel for water dripping. *World J Surg.* 1999;23:1032–1037.
5. Yamamoto J, Kosuge T, Shimada K, Yamasaki S, Takayama T, Makuuchi M. Anterior transhepatic approach for isolated resection of the caudate lobe of the liver. *World J Surg.* 1999;23:97–101.
6. Weber JC, Navarra G, Jiao LR, Nicholls JP, Jensen SL, Habib NA. New technique for liver resection using heat coagulative necrosis. *Ann Surg.* 2002;236:560–563.
7. Gazelle GS, Goldberg SN, Solbiati L, Livraghi T. Tumor ablation with radio-frequency energy. *Radiology.* 2000;217:633–646.
8. Livraghi T, Goldberg SN, Lazzaroni S, Meloni F, Ierace T, Solbiati L, Gazelle GS. Hepatocellular carcinoma: radio-frequency ablation of medium and large lesions. *Radiology.* 2000;214:761–768.

9. Rossi S, Garbagnati F, Lencioni R, Allgaier HP, Marchiano A, Fornari F, Quaretti P, Tolla GD, Ambrosi C, Mazzaferro V, Blum HE, Bartolozzi C. Percutaneous radio-frequency thermal ablation of nonresectable hepatocellular carcinoma after occlusion of tumor blood supply. *Radiology.* 2000;217:119–126.

10. Solbiati L, Goldberg SN, Ierace T, Dellanoce M, Livraghi T, Gazelle GS. Radio-frequency ablation of hepatic metastases: postprocedural assessment with a US microbubble contrast agent—early experience. *Radiology.* 1999;211:643–649.

11. Steiner P, Botnar R, Dubno B, Zimmermann GG, Gazelle GS, Debatin JF. Radio-frequency-induced thermoablation: monitoring with T1-weighted and proton-frequency-shift MR imaging in an interventional 0.5-T environment. *Radiology.* 1998;206:803–810.

12. Ahmed M, Goldberg SN. Radiofrequency tissue ablation: principles and techniques. In: Ellis LM, Curley SA, Tanabe KK, eds. Radiofrequency Ablation for Cancer. New York: Springer Verlag; 2003.

13. Larson TR, Bostwick DG, Gorcia A. Temperature-correlated histopathologic changes following microwave thermoablation of obstructive tissue in patients with benign prostatic hyperplasia. *Urology.* 1996;47:463–469.

14. Hansler J, Neuretier D, Strobel D, Mutter D, BernatikT, Hahn EG, Becker D. Cellular and vascular reactions in the liver to radio-frequency thermo-ablation with wet needle applicators. *Eur Surg Res.* 2002;34:357–363.

Islet Cell Allotransplantation: Development of a Clinical Programme in West London

VASSILIOS E. PAPALOIS

St. Mary's and the Hammersmith Hospitals, London, UK

1.   INTRODUCTION

The purpose of this research study is to isolate a high yield of viable purified islets from human pancreases under sterile conditions. If this is successful, then the researchers will apply to the Department of Health and the United Kingdom Transplant Support Service Authority for permission to perform islet transplantation in humans for the treatment of insulin dependent diabetes mellitus.

2.   SCIENTIFIC BACKGROUND OF STUDY

Since January 1995, patients with type I diabetes and end stage renal failure have been treated in our unit with combined kidney/pancreas transplantation. In addition, type I diabetics with great difficulties in controlling their diabetes but with good kidney function are offered the opportunity of a pancreas transplant alone. The results for long term patient and graft survival in our institution and around the world have been very good. However, pancreas transplantation remains a major procedure with not negligible morbidity.

The first advantage of islet transplantation is that it is a simple procedure that does not require surgical intervention. It can be done radiologically via percutaneous intraperitoneal or intraportal injection. The second advantage is that the failure of the transplant is not associated with morbidity. Finally, the transplant can be repeated many times without significant discomfort to the patient.

During the last 25 years, many clinical islet transplants have been performed but the results have been very disappointing. There are three main reasons for this: difficulty in extracting a high yield of viable islets from human pancreases, islet toxicity of the immunosuppressive drugs, and lack of reliable markers for early diagnosis of rejection. Recently there have been many significant improvements in the field of islet transplantation. The first was the development of a semi-automated method for islet extraction, which has tripled the number of viable islets that can be isolated from a human pancreas. Secondly, there are some immunosuppressive regimens that avoid completely the use of steroids (with their well known diabetogenic effects) and that focus on the use of low dosages of Tacrolimus and Rapamycin. The issue of early detection of rejection is still to be solved.

The progress in the field of islet transplantation is reflected in the recent results published by Shapiro et al.[1] This group reported a total of seven patients transplanted with islets

89

N. A. Habib and R. Canelo (eds.), Liver and Pancreatic Diseases Management, 89–93.
© 2006 *Springer. Printed in The Netherlands.*

between March 1999 and January 2000. The median graft survival (insulin dependence) was 11.9 months (duration 4.4–14.9). The updated experience (May 2003) from the same group,[2] showed that for 43 recipients of islets transplants the overall 1 and 3 year graft survival (insulin independence) was 80 and 55%, respectively. These results have encouraged many groups around the world (including ours) to pursue clinical islet transplantation programmes.

Our unit has demonstrated a research interest in islet transplantation since 1995, focusing on islet xenotransplantation. The pig has always been considered the most suitable donor for a potential animal to human xenotransplantation. Over the years we have performed multiple digestions of porcine pancreases and isolations of islets. We have identified xenoantigens expressed on pig islets that are recognized in humans during the process of hyperacute rejection. We have also developed methods for eliminating the expression of those xenoantigens. Our laboratory (the Brent Laboratory, 4th Floor Clarence Memorial Wing, St Mary's Hospital) has all the state-of-the-art technology for islet isolation from human pancreases. Between June 2000 and June 2001, we have extracted islets from 25 pig pancreases in order to optimize our methodology prior to proceeding to islet isolation from human pancreases. We are able to extract more than 500,000 viable islets from each pig pancreas under entirely sterile conditions. Because of these highly successful results we decided to proceed to isolating islets from human pancreases.

3.   PROTOCOL OF THE STUDY

We obtained permission from the London Multicentre Research Ethics Committee as well as from all the North Thames Local Research Ethics Committees to proceed with procuring pancreases from cadaveric donors in the North Thames Region in order to isolate islets. The stages of our protocol are as follows:

1. When a donor becomes available in the North Thames Transplant Region, the Regional Transplant Coordinator inform us. Currently, only donors less than 50 years old are being considered for donation of the pancreas for whole organ transplant. If the donor is more than 50 years old, or if the donor is less than 50 years old but the pancreas cannot be used for whole organ transplant (unavailability of a suitable recipient, inflammation, or trauma of the pancreas), the Coordinator presents the outline of our project to the donor family and they are asked if they want to offer the pancreas for research.

2. If the pancreas is offered for research, a surgical team from our unit goes to the hospital where the retrieval will take place and will join the teams that will procure other organs for whole organ transplantation. Our team has all the surgical equipment, preservation solutions, and storage equipment that are necessary to procure and store safely the pancreas.

3. The multiorgan procurement proceeds according to the standard protocol used by the teams in the North Thames Region: after opening of the chest and the abdomen, meticulous dissection of the organs to be retrieved is performed. Following this, intravascular flushing takes place and replacement of the blood of the donor with preservation solution. The final step is the meticulous removal of the organs that are

going to be used for transplantation. Our team intervenes only when the retrieval of the organs for whole organ transplant has been completed. The pancreatic gland is detached from the surrounding tissue by using sharp dissection. The duodenum is also procured en bloc with the pancreas. By applying the GIA 60 stapling/dividing device twice (just after the pylorus and close to the ligament of Treitz), the duodenum is separated from the rest of the bowel and is procured with the pancreas. This is necessary in order to be able to identify the ampulla of Vater and via that the pancreatic duct. The pancreatic duct is used to inject the enzyme collagenase into the pancreas in order to be able to digest it and isolate the islets. The procurement of the pancreas takes approximately 15 min.

4. The pancreatic graft is placed by our team into a sterile bag containing 500 cc University of Wisconsin solution. This solution has been proved to be the best solution for preservation of the pancreatic graft. Following the placement of the pancreas, this bag is tightly closed and is placed into another sterile bag which will also be tightly closed. The two bags containing the pancreatic graft are placed into a special container and they are covered completely by ice.

5. The pancreas is transferred to the Brent Laboratory, 4th Floor, Clarence Memorial Wing at St Mary's Hospital and is placed in the culture room.

6. The pancreas is then transferred into a laminar flow hood (which has an entirely sterile environment) and is placed into a sterile kidney dish into a mixture of University of Wisconsin solution and ice.

7. Two members of our research team dissect the pancreas. These two researchers are scrubbed and they wear hats, masks, as well as sterile gowns and gloves.

8. All the fatty tissue, vessels, lymphatic, and ganglionic tissue is removed from the pancreatic gland. By opening the duodenum of the pancreatic graft, the ampulla of Vater is identified and by this the pancreatic duct is identified. Following this, the duodenum is removed and the pancreatic duct is cannulated with a size 6 French cannula. By encircling the pancreatic duct with a 2/0 silk tie, the cannula is secured.

9. Hank's solution (500 cc) containing collagenase-P (concentration 1 mg/ml) is injected via the cannula into the pancreatic duct.

10. Following that, the pancreas is digested by using the Recordi semi-automated method. All the devices that are being used for this method are sterilized prior to the digestion and are placed into the laminar flow hood. The chamber is filled with Hank's solution containing antibiotics (Penicillin 50 IU/ml, Streptomycin 50 µg/ml, Gentamicin 50 µg/ml, and Fluconazole 25 µg/ml). The temperature inside the chamber can be monitored at any time by a temperature sensor which is attached to it. The chamber is connected to a closed circuit, which is attached to: (a) a pump; (b) a water bath; (c) a cannula. The pump is used in order to facilitate the re-circulation of the Hank's solution within the closed circuit and the chamber. The water bath is used in order to increase the temperature within the circuit and the chamber up to 37 °C. The cannula is used in order to obtain samples from the circuit, as well as for draining the chamber and the circuit at the end of the digestion. By turning the pump on, circulation of the Hank's solution within the system starts, and as soon as the temperature of the solution reaches 37 °C, the collagenase which is injected into the pancreas is activated. Gradually the collagenase digests

the pancreas into very small pieces of tissue. Due to the presence of a filter in the outflow of the chamber, only the islets and part of the exocrine tissue can go out of the chamber and into the closed circuit. As soon as the tissue is visualized to come out of the chamber and into the circuit, the cannula is opened and a small sample is obtained. The sample is then stained with Dithizone, which is a special stain that can be obtained only from the islets. The sample is observed under the microscope to confirm the presence of the islets. Similar samples are obtained at intervals of 5 min. As soon as the pancreatic tissue represents approximately 50–160% of the tissue of the sample, the digestion is considered to be completed. Following this, the cannula of the system is opened and the Hank's solution containing the islet tissue mixed with exocrine tissue is collected into sterile bottles containing cold Hank's solution with antibiotics at the concentrations previously described.

11. The bottles containing the mixed islet and exocrine tissue are placed in the centrifuge and they will are spun down in 2000 rpm for 5 min as a first effort to separate the islet tissue from the exocrine tissue. The same procedure is repeated 3 times.

12. The supernate from the last spin is collected in sterile bottles and an effort is made to separate almost completely the islet tissue from the exocrine tissue in order to obtain and almost completely purified islet preparation.

    The polysaccharide dextran is mixed with Hank's solution in order to prepare four different concentrations: (a) 50 ml 31% dextran, (b) 50 ml 28% dextran, (c) 50 ml 23% dextran, and (d) 50 ml 11% dextran. The pH of all these solutions is 7.4. The supernate containing the islet tissue and exocrine tissue is mixed at the bottom of the conical tube with concentration (a) of dextran. The concentrations (b), (c), and (d) are then applied gently on top of the bottom layer containing the dextran with the islet tissue. The conical tube is spun down at initially 400 rpm for 4 min and then at 2,000 rpm for 16 min. At the end of this procedure, the islet tissue is separated from the exocrine tissue and should be in the interface between the top concentration (11%) and the one below it (23%). Most of the exocrine tissue should be settled at the bottom concentration (31%) and the concentration of 28%.

13. The islet tissue is collected from the interface of the top two layers and is then mixed with 50 ml Hank's solution and it is spun down at 2,000 rpm for 5 min in order to separate the islet tissue from the polysaccharide dextran. The supernate is collected and is again mixed with Hank's solution and spun down at 2,000 rpm for 5 min for two more times. The last supernate is collected and is placed into a sterile flask containing 200 cc RPMI culture medium containing antibiotics. Two samples are obtained at this point from the mixture of islets with RPMI. The first sample is approximately 1 ml of tissue, which is stained with Dithizone and observed under the microscope. In this 1 ml of tissue, the amount of islets present, as well as their purity (percentage of islets in the whole tissue present) is counted. Knowing how many islets are in 1 ml of the mixture of islet cells and RPMI, it is easy to calculate the total number of islets isolated from a certain pancreas. For the last 10 isolatio, steps 13 and 14 are being done by using the Cobe 2991 automated cell separator.

14. Two samples from this preparation of islets and RPMI are sent also to Microbiology in order to be examined for possible presence of bacteria or fungi.

15. The preparation of islets and RPMI are then equally separated into two flasks. The first one is placed in an incubator in order to culture the islet cells, and the second one is used in order to test the viability of the islet cells.

In the flask that is selected in order to test islet viability, into the RPMI solution containing the islets, approximately 20 ml containing 50% dextrose are added. The presence of dextrose stimulates the islets to produce insulin. The islets are incubated with dextrose for approximately 2 h. At the end of this procedure, the content of the flask is placed into a sterile conical tube and is spun down at 2000 rpm for 5 min. The supernate is collected and the presence of insulin is estimated by using the gamma counter. The flask containing the islets is kept under sterile conditions in the incubator for approximately two weeks. At the end of these 2 weeks, a new sample is sent to Microbiology to check for the presence of bacteria or fungi in order to confirm the sterility of the islet preparation.

4.   RESULTS

From October 2001 to October 2003, we have isolated islets from 23 pancreases. The yield varied from 70,000 to 240,000 islet equivalents (>150,000 for the last five isolations) with >80% purity. The islets remained sterile and they were insulin producing.

5.   FUTURE

Our very good results allow us to believe that, after obtaining permission from the St. Mary's Local Research Ethics Committee we will initiate a clinical islet transplantation programme in early 2004.

REFERENCES

1. Shapiro J, Lakey J, RyanE, et al. Islet transplantation in seven patients with type 1 diabetes mellitus using a glucocorticoid free immunosuppressive regimen. *N Engl J Med.* 2000;343(4):230–238.
2. Shapiro J, Ryan E, Paty B, et al. Three year follow up in clinical islet alone transplant with the Edmonton protocol and preliminary impact of Infliximab and Campath-1H. *Am J Transplant.* 2000;3 (Suppl. 5):296.

Whole Organ Pancreas Transplantation

NADEY S. HAKIM

Transplant Unit, St Mary's Hospital, Praed Street, London W2 1NY, UK

1.   INTRODUCTION

The syndrome of type I insulin-dependent diabetes mellitus (IDDM) includes not only abnormal glucose metabolism but also specific microvascular complications such as retinopathy, nephropathy, and neuropathy. Diabetes mellitus is currently the leading cause of kidney failure and blindness in adults, the number one disease cause of amputations and impotence, and one of the leading chronic diseases of childhood associated with poor quality of life.

The aim of pancreas and islet transplantation is to establish the same status of glucose control that is provided by endogenous secretion of insulin from a healthy native pancreas in order to improve the quality of life and ameliorate secondary diabetic complications in patients with IDDM.

The first pancreas transplant in a human was performed by Kelly et al. on 16 December 1966 at the University of Minnesota.[1]

Islet transplantation is, theoretically, an ideal solution for patients with IDDM since it is not a major procedure, it can be performed radiologically and can be repeated several times without any major discomfort to the patient. Islet transplantation in humans has been performed systematically since 1974 and, as with pancreas transplantation, the University of Minnesota pioneered the field.[2] However, despite tedious experimental and clinical efforts over the past 25 years, long-term and consistent insulin independence has not yet been achieved.

2.   INDICATIONS

Pancreas transplantation is indicated for patients with IDDM and additional selection criteria are listed in Table 1. Patient selection is aided by comprehensive multidisciplinary pre-transplant evaluation with additional work up according to the specific problems of each patient. The evaluation initially confirms the diagnosis of IDDM, establishes the absence of any exclusion criteria, determines the patient's ability to tolerate a major operation (based primarily on the patient's cardiovascular status), and documents end-stage organ complications for future tracking following transplantation.

In a suitable candidate, the evaluation is also needed to determine the type of pancreas transplantation, based mainly on the degree of nephropathy. The degree of renal dysfunction (creatinine clearance below 20 ml/min) is used to select patients for simultaneous pancreas—kidney transplantation (SPK) versus pancreas transplant alone (PTA) (creatinine clearance

N. A. Habib and R. Canelo (eds.), Liver and Pancreatic Diseases Management, 95–105.
© *2006 Springer. Printed in The Netherlands.*

Table 1. Exclusion and inclusion criteria

Exclusion criteria
  Insufficient cardiovascular reserve
    Angiography indicating non-correctable coronary artery disease
    Ejection fraction below 50%
    Recent myocardial infarction
  Current significant
    Psychiatric illness
    Psychological instability
    Drug or alcohol abuse
    Non-compliance with treatment
  Active infection
  Malignancy
  Lack of well-defined secondary diabetic complications
  Extreme obesity (>130% of ideal body weight)
Inclusion criteria
  Presence of IDDM
  Well-defined secondary diabetic complications
  Ability to withstand
    Surgery
    Immunosuppression
  Psychological suitability
  Good understanding of
    Therapeutic nature of pancreas transplantation
    Need for long-term immunosuppression and follow-up
    Criteria for SPK, PTA, and PAK (Table 2)

---

above 70 ml/min). A third option is to transplant a pancreas after a kidney (PAK) in patients with IDDM who have already had a kidney transplant and who meet the criteria for pancreas transplantation. The criteria for SPK, PTA, and PAK transplants are summarized in Table 2.

3.   RECIPIENT OPERATION

The majority of pancreas transplants is performed in conjunction with a kidney transplant from the same donor through a midline incision intraperitoneal approach. The same approach is used for PTA and PAK transplants. The surgical approach to pancreas transplantation is similar to that for the kidney in many aspects. The pancreas is directed with the head towards the pelvis and, usually, the graft vessels are anastomosed end-to-side to the recipient common or external iliac vessels using 5–0 Prolene suture for the venous and 6–0 Prolene suture for the arterial anastomosis. If possible, the vessels are anastomosed to the right iliac vessels of the recipient, which are more superficial compared to the left iliac vessels. This minimizes the chances of post-transplant graft thrombosis. In order to prevent thrombosis of the portal vein of the pancreatic graft, it is important to ligate and

Table 2. Criteria for SPK, PTA, and PAK transplants

Criteria for SPK
    Diabetic nephropathy: creatinine clearance <20 ml/min
    Patient on dialysis or very close to starting dialysis
    Failure of previous renal allograft
Criteria for PTA
    The presence of two or more diabetic complications:
        Proliferative retinopathy
        Early nephropathy; creatinine clearance > 70 ml/min,
proteinuria >150 mg/24 h but <3 g/24 h
        Presence of overt peripheral or autonomic neuropathy
        Vasculopathy with accelerated atherosclerosis
    Hyperlabile diabetes with:
        Severe episodes of ketoacidosis
        Severe and frequent episodes of hypoglycemia
        Hypoglycemia unawareness
        Severe and frequent infections
        Impairment of quality of life
Criteria for PAK
    Patients with stable function of previous renal allograft
that meet the criteria for PTA

divide the internal iliac vein in order to free the common and external iliac veins prior to the anastomosis with the portal vein. This type of venous anastomosis results in systemic drainage of the venous outflow of the pancreatic graft. More recently, the University of Tennessee[3] has introduced a portal drainage technique where the pancreas is placed head up and the portal vein anastomosed to one of the mesenteric veins. This achieves a more physiological drainage into the portal circulation. This technique is possibly associated with a higher rate of technical complications while there is no clear evidence that it has better metabolic results. The only possible advantage of portal drainage is the absence of systemic hyperinsulinemia which is characteristic of systemic drainage.

Several surgical techniques have been used to manage the exocrine secretions of the pancreatic graft, including urinary drainage, enteric drainage, or polymer injection. Urinary drainage is currently the most popular, but enteric drainage has recently regained popularity. Duct injection is becoming less and less popular even in the European centers where it was first introduced.[4]

3.1.   Urinary Drainage

The creation of the duodenocystostomy starts by opening the bladder anteriorly and longitudinally. The anastomosis is done either manually or using a stapler, the latter being the most popular technique. The major advantage of this technique is the ability to detect pancreas rejection episodes early (before hyperglycemia) by monitoring urinary amylase. It is, however, associated with significant morbidity, including duodenal leaks, cystitis, urethritis, reflux pancreatitis, dehydration, acidosis, and electrolyte abnormalities.[5]

3.2.   Enteric Drainage

The duodenum is anastomosed side-to-side in two layers to a loop of proximal ileum while avoiding any tension. The distal duodenum is closed as described earlier. The enteric drainage of exocrine secretions is more physiological in view of the bowel reabsorption. However, urinary amylase cannot be used as a rejection maker and eventual leaks can lead to severe complications.

3.3.   Duct Injection

The injection of polymer into the main pancreatic duct is a very simple and fast technique, which leads eventually to the atrophy of the exocrine portion of the pancreas. Unfortunately it can lead too to the atrophy of the endocrine tissue, resulting in graft failure.

4.   IMMUNOSUPPRESSION

Optimal immunosuppressive strategies in pancreas transplantation aim at achieving effective control of rejection while minimizing injury to the allograft as well as risk to the patient. Until recently a standard immunosuppressive protocol consisted of cyclosporine (cyclosporin A), prednisone, and azathioprine combined with an induction course of anti-T cell monoclonal or polyclonal antibody (antilymphocyte globulin (ALG), antithymocyte globulin (ATG), or OKT3). Tacrolimus has replaced cyclosporine in 20% of centers and more recently mycophenolate mofetil (MMF) has been used instead of azathioprine.[3] Studies have demonstrated higher patient and graft survival rates. Transplantation requires a lifelong commitment to immunosuppression. However, most patients find it easier to adjust to their immunosuppressive medications than to insulin, dietary, and activity restrictions.

5.   RESULTS

From December 1966 up to date over 16,000 pancreas transplants have been performed worldwide. The latest publication of the International Pancreas Transplant Register (IPTR) data include 8,800 pancreas transplants that had been performed from December 1966 to November 1996, including more than 6,400 from the U.S.A. and more than 2,300 from other countries.[6] Most of those transplants (86%) were SPK, 8% were PAK, and 5% were PTA. Outside the U.S.A. most were performed in Europe (91%). The leading country was France (19%), followed by Germany (16%), Sweden (10%), and Spain (7%).

For the 4,592 bladder-drained pancreas transplants performed in the U.S.A. between October 1987 and November 1996, the patient survival rates at 1, 2, 3, and 5 years were 92%, 89%, 86%, and 81%, respectively. Graft survival rates at 1, 2, 3, and 5 years were 76%, 71%, 67%, and 61% for all cases. When only the 4,062 technically successful cases were considered, the 1-, 2-, 3- and 5-year graft survival was 85%, 81%, 76%, and 72%, respectively. When the same data were analyzed by recipient category, the 1-, 2-, 3- and 5-year patient survival was 92%, 89%, 86% and 81% for SPK ($n = 3,989$), 91%, 87%,

82%, and 74% for PAK ($n = 375$), and 90%, 88%, 86%, and 81% for PTA ($n = 229$), respectively. The patient survival rate was not significantly different ($p > 0.22$) between the three recipient categories. For the same period, graft survival at 1, 2, 3, and 5 years was 79%, 75%, 71%, and 65% for SPK, 58%, 45%, 38%, and 27% for PAK, and 56%, 48%, 40%, and 32% for PTA, respectively. Graft survival was significantly different between the three categories ($p = 0.0001$). The outcome was significantly better for SPK than for PTA, but there was no difference between PTA and PAK ($p = 0.83$). The technical failure rate was lower in the SPK category compared to PTA. There was no significant difference for 1-year graft survival rates for primary versus retransplants in the SPK (79% vs. 77%, $p > 0.10$) and PTA (57% vs. 51%, $p > 0.8$) categories. In contrast, for PAK transplants, 1-year graft survival was higher in primary transplants than in retransplants (62% vs. 47%, $p < 0.0001$).

The results of pancreas transplantation in European and other non-U.S. centers are comparable to those in the U.S.A. One-year patient survival for SPK in the U.S.A., Europe, and other countries was 92%, 91%, and 86% respectively ($p = 0.08$). One-year graft survival for bladder-drained SPK in the U.S.A., Europe, and other countries was 79%, 73%, and 70%, respectively ($p < 0.08$). Likewise, 1-year graft survival for enterically drained SPK in the U.S.A., Europe, and other countries was 72%, 63%, and 72%, respectively ($p > 0.7$).

5.1. Effect of Pancreas Transplantation on Secondary Complications of IDDM

The results of patient and graft survival after pancreatic transplantation have significantly improved in the last decade. Pancreas transplantation is not a lifesaving procedure, and the assessment of its effect on the progress of the secondary diabetic complications as well as the overall quality of life of pancreas transplant recipients is of great importance.

One major problem in studying the effects of pancreas transplantation on halting or, even more, reversing the progress of secondary diabetic complications is that many pancreas transplant recipients have end-stage degenerative diabetic complications, for which there is no hope for improvement. In addition, since the majority of pancreas transplants is performed simultaneously with a kidney, it is difficult to differentiate and attribute any positive development after SPK to the effect of the normal status of glucose metabolism rather than to the corrected uremia. Finally, most of the studies that deal with the effect of pancreas transplantation on diabetic complications are not multicenter prospective randomized trials with large numbers of patients and long-term follow-up from which reliable conclusions could be reached.

5.2. Retinopathy

There is some controversy on the effect of pancreas transplantation on diabetic retinopathy. Most of these studies were performed in patients already affected by proliferative retinopathy. In one of these studies with follow-up of 4 or more years after transplantation, stabilization of retinopathy was observed, more than that observed in patients followed for the same period of time but whose pancreas transplants had failed.[7] In another study two groups of diabetic patients were included: in the first group the patients underwent SPK and in the second a kidney transplant alone.[8] The status of diabetic retinopathy remained unchanged in 88% and 90% of these patients, respectively. The results were similar in another study performed in diabetic patients who underwent PTA; the post-transplant euglycemia did not change the course of diabetic retinopathy.[9]

5.3.   Nephropathy

In one study of diabetic patients who underwent pancreas transplantation after having had a successful kidney transplant, it was demonstrated that pancreas transplantation prevents, to some extent, recurrence of diabetic nephropathy and that the diabetic glomerular lesions were less severe compared to diabetic patients that underwent a kidney transplant alone.[10] However, studies performed on patients who received a PTA showed that the diabetic glomerular lesions did not improve even after several years of achieving an insulin-independent euglycemic state with pancreas transplantation.[11]

5.4.   Neuropathy

A number of studies have reported improvements in both motor and sensory nerve function as assessed by nerve conduction velocity in SPK compared both to recipients of kidney transplant alone and patients with pancreatic graft failure.[12,13] These studies clearly demonstrated that although the correction of uremia by a simultaneous kidney transplant, or a kidney transplant alone, significantly improves motor and sensory nerve conduction, the presence of a pancreatic graft has an additional and important positive effect in improving peripheral neuropathy. Studies of the effect of pancreas transplantation on autonomic neuropathy were performed in PTA and compared to non-transplanted patients or patients after pancreas graft failure.[14] The cardiorespiratory reflexes were evaluated in these patients and analyzed in relation to the survival rate. These studies demonstrated that PTA with a functioning pancreatic graft had better survival rates compared to recipients with a failed pancreatic graft as well as compared to diabetics who were not transplanted. However, other studies of autonomic function following pancreas transplantation are less clear. In some, pancreas transplantation was associated with greater improvement in autonomic symptoms, even if they were accompanied by little objective evidence.[15,16]

6.   QUALITY OF LIFE AFTER PANCREAS TRANSPLANTATION

Patient and graft survival rates, the incidence of morbidity, and the effect of transplantation on the secondary diabetic complications are definitely of great significance in evaluating the results. What is perhaps of even greater significance is the effect that pancreas transplantation has on the overall quality of life of diabetic patients. The effect on the quality of life is important for the evaluation of all modern therapeutic interventions, but it is even more important in the case of a non-lifesaving organ transplant which carries a non-negligible risk and involves many social and financial aspects. It is encouraging that it is in the field of quality of life that many studies agree that pancreas transplantation has a very positive effect.

A detailed study evaluated the effect of pancreas transplantation on many different aspects of life quality of 157 diabetic patients.[17] The results indicated a much better quality of life (satisfaction with physical capacity as well as leisure time activities) in recipients of SPK compared to pre-transplant pre-dialysis diabetic patients.

In an interesting study, authors reported on the benefit of SPK compared to kidney transplant alone.[18] Of all SPK, 90% had full-time occupations post-transplant compared to 50% of recipients of kidney transplant alone. In addition, lost working days decreased by 44% compared to the pre-transplant situation in the SPK, whereas in recipients of kidneys only there was no change. Furthermore, SPK achieved a better quality of life in physical well-being, sole functioning, and perception of self.

In another extensive analysis, 131 recipients of pancreatic transplant 1–11 years post-transplant were studied.[19] Patients with functioning pancreatic grafts were compared with recipients with failed grafts who had good kidney function. The recipients with functioning graft compared to recipients with non-functioning grafts reported more satisfaction with the overall quality of life (68% vs. 48%), felt healthier (89% vs. 25%), and were able to care for themselves and their daily activities (78% vs. 56%).

In a prospective study with 1-year follow-up using the Medical Outcome Study Health Survey 36-Item Short Form (SF-36) and comparing SPK recipients to kidney transplants alone and IDDM patients who did not receive a transplant, improvement of general health perception, social function, vitality, and pain was seen in both transplanted groups. However, physical limitations improved only in SPK recipients.[20] In addition, financial situation, physical capacity, occupational status, sexual, and leisure time activities improved significantly for SPK recipients.[21]

7.   ISLET TRANSPLANTATION

7.1.   Advantages and Problems of Islet Transplantation

As previously mentioned, islet transplantation is, in theory, an ideal solution for patients with IDDM since it is not a major procedure, it can be performed radiologically and can be repeated several times without any major discomfort to the patient. Unfortunately there are many problems related to islet transplantation, the most difficult being the availability of human organs for islet allotransplantation. Indeed, of approximately 5,000 donors available each year in the U.S.A., only a small proportion is suitable for pancreas or islet transplantation, and most of those are used for whole organ pancreas transplantation. The technique for islet isolation has to be meticulous in order to obtain a good yield of viable islets. There is great difficulty in early detection of islet allograft rejection, even when they are transplanted simultaneously with a kidney. Finally, the islets are very sensitive to the currently used drugs in the standardized immunosuppressive regimens such as steroids, cyclosporine, and tacrolimus.

7.2.   Human Islet Allografts

After many years of research, it was only in the late 1980s that it became possible to perform islet allotransplants with some success. The islets obtained from cadaveric donors were transplanted into the liver via the portal vein. Initial results were encouraging, but were later disappointing as it became obvious that most recipients remained hyperglycemic. By the end of 1995, 270 patients with IDDM, who received adult islet allografts were reported to the International Islet Transplant Registry (IITR)[22] Of these, only 27 (10%) became insulin independent for more than 1 week, 14 (5%) were insulin independent for more than 1 week, 14 (5%) were insulin independent for more than 1 year, and 1 patient was insulin independent for more than 4 years. Factors related to short-term insulin independence are detailed in Table 3. In addition to the classical immunosuppressive protocols, induction therapy with 15-deoxyspergualin is an important factor for achieving relatively long-term insulin independence. The reason is the ability of 15-deoxyspergualin to minimize the macrophage-mediated attack that islet allografts (as well as autografts) undergo post-transplant and which causes the phenomenon of islet primary non-function.[23] Although the IITR results for long-term insulin independence are not good, it is important to emphasize that many of the insulin-dependent islet recipients have had persisting C-peptide secretion, a reduction of insulin dose, and improvement in stability of glucose control, which correlated with less dangerous hypoglycemic episodes. This means that it is possible for some of the transplanted islets to survive a long time with improvements in islet isolation techniques, as well as improvements in detection of rejection and immunosuppression, long-term insulin independence with islet allotransplantation might become a reality.

Patients who underwent pancreatectomy and hepatectomy for extensive abdominal cancer followed by simultaneous islet and liver grafts had very good islet function posttransplant.[22] Indeed, 9 out of 15 (60%) became insulin independent. Ultimately all patients succumbed to their malignancy, one of them having remained insulin independent for 5 years until her death. The reasons for these better results compared to the results of islet transplants in patients with IDDM are not clear. A possible explanation is that islets only had to overcome allograft rejection and not the autoimmune response associated with IDDM. The fact that these patients had cancer could have compromised their immunity and finally the simultaneous liver transplant could have had a protective element.

Table 3. Factors related with insulin independence after islet allotransplantation

---

Presentation time <8 h
Transplantation of >6,000 islet equivalents (number of islets
    if all had a diameter of 150 μm/kg of body weight)
Transplantation into the liver via the portal vein
Induction immunosuppression with anti-T cell agents and
    15-deoxyspergualin

7.3.   The Future of Pancreas and Islet Transplantation

The advances in immunosuppressive strategies and diagnostic technology will only enhance the already good results achieved with pancreas transplantation. Further documentation of the long-term benefits and effects of pancreas transplantation may lead to wider availability and acceptance. Prevention of rejection and effective control with earlier diagnosis may soon permit solitary pancreas transplantation to become an acceptable option in diabetic patients without advanced secondary complications or diabetes. During the past decade, significant advances have been achieved in islet transplantation.[24] The success of islet autografts indicates that successful engraftment and function of human islets is possible and, with some advancements in rejection monitoring and immunosuppression, results of islet allotransplantation will also improve. The recent developments in the field of islet xenotransplantation and microencapsulation enhance the belief that islet transplantation will become an ideal option for the treatment of IDDM. Currently, however, islet transplantation cannot compete with the results obtained with whole organ pancreas transplantation. Therefore, while continuing with the tedious but promising research work to improve the results of islet transplantation, every patient with IDDM who meets the criteria should be offered the option of pancreas transplantation.

8.   KEY POINTS FOR CLINICAL PRACTICE

1. The aim of pancreas and islet transplantation is to establish the same status of glucose control that is provided by endogenous secretion of insulin from a healthy native pancreas in order to improve the quality of life and ameliorate secondary diabetic complications in patients with IDDM.
2. Optimal immunosuppressive strategies in pancreas transplantation aim at achieving effective control of rejection while minimizing injury to the allograft as well as risk to the patient.
3. Pancreas transplantation is not a lifesaving procedure, and the assessment of its effect on the progress of the secondary diabetic complications as well as the overall quality of life of pancreas transplant recipients is of great importance.
4. Pancreas transplantation prevents, to some extent, recurrence of diabetic nephropathy and that the diabetic glomerular lesions were less severe compared to diabetic patients that underwent a kidney transplant alone.
5. A number of studies have reported improvements in both motor and sensory nerve function as assessed by nerve conduction velocity in SPK compared both to recipients of kidney transplant alone and patients with pancreatic graft failure.
6. A much better quality of life (satisfaction with physical capacity as well as leisure time activities) in recipients of SPK compared to pre-transplant pre-dialysis diabetic patients.

    The technique for islet isolation has to be meticulous in order to obtain a good yield of viable islets. There is great difficulty in early detection of islet allograft rejection, even when they are transplanted simultaneously with a kidney.

7. While continuing with the tedious but promising research work to improve the results of islet transplantation, every patient with IDDM who meets the criteria should be offered the option of pancreas transplantation.

REFERENCES

1. Kelly W, Lillehi R, Merkel F. Allotransplantation of the pancreas and duodenum along with the kidney in diabetic nephropathy. *Surgery.* 1967;61:827–835.
2. Najarian J, Sutherland DER, Steffes M. Isolation of human islets of Langerhans for transplantation. *Transplant Proc.* 1975;7:611–613.
3. Stratta R. Pancreas transplantation in the 1990s. In: Hakim NS, Stratta R, Dubernard J-M, eds. Proceedings of the Second British Symposium on Pancreas and Islet Transplantation (ICSS 232). London: Royal Society of Medicine; 1998: 103–121.
4. Dubernard JM, Tajra LC, Dawahra M, et al. Improving morbidity rates of reno-pancreatic transplantation by modification of the technique. In: Hakim NS, Stratta R, Dubernard J-M, eds. Proceedings of the Second British Symposium on Pancreas and Islet Transplantation (ICSS, 232). London: Royal Society of Medicine.
5. Hakim NS, Gruessner A, Papalois VE, et al. Duodenal complications in bladder-drained pancreas transplants. *Surgery.* 1997;121(6):618–624.
6. Gruessner A, Sutherland DER, Goetz F, et al. Pancreas transplantation in the United States (US) and non-US as reported to the United Network for Organ Sharing (UNOS) and the International Pancreas Transplant Registry (IPTR). In: Terasaki P, Cecka J, eds. Clinical Transplants 1996. Los Angeles: LA Tissue Typing Laboratory; 1996: 47–67.
7. Bandello F, Vigano C, et al. Influence of successful pancreatorenal transplantation on diabetic retinopathy: a 20 cases report. *Diabetologia.* 1991;34 (suppl 1):92–94.
8. Caldara R, Bandello F, Vigano C, et al. Influence of successful pancreatorenal transplantation on diabetic nephropathy. *Transplant Proc.* 1994;26:490.
9. Ransay RC, Frederich CB, Sutherland DER, et al. Progression of diabetic retinopathy after pancreas transplantation for insulin-dependent diabetes mellitus. *N Engl J Med.* 1988;318:208–214.
10. Billus RW, Mauer SM, Sutherland DER, et al. The effect of pancreas transplantation on the glomerular structure of renal allografts in patients with insulin-dependent diabetes. *N Engl J Med.* 1989;321:80–85.
11. Fioretto P, Mauer SM, Bilou RW, et al. Effects of pancreas transplantation on glomerular structure in insulin-dependent diabetic patients with their own kidneys. *Lancet.* 1993;342:1193–1196.
12. Comi G, Galardi G, Amadio S, et al. Neurophysiological study of the effect of combined kidney and pancreas transplantation on diabetic neuropathy: a 2-year follow-up evaluation. *Diabetologia.* 1991;34(suppl I):103–107.
13. Solders G, Tyden G, Persson A, et al. Improvement of nerve conduction in diabetic nephropathy. *Diabetes.* 1992;41:946–951.
14. Navarro X, Kennedy WR, Goetz FGC, et al. Influence of pancreas transplantation on cardiorespiratory reflexes, nerve conduction, and mortality in diabetes mellitus. *Diabetes.* 1990;39:802–806.
15. Nusser J, Scheuer R, Abendroth D, et al. Effect of pancreatic transplantation and/or renal transplantation on diabetic autonomic neuropathy. *Diabetologia.* 1991;34 (suppl I):118–120.
16. Hathaway DK, Abell T, Cardoso S, et al. Improvement in autonomic and gastric function following pancreas—kidney versus kidney-alone transplantation and the correlation with quality of life. *Transplantation.* 1994;57:816–822.
17. La Rocca E, Secchi A, Galardi G, et al. Kidney and pancreas transplantation improves hypertension in type I diabetic patients. Abstract book, 7th Congress of the European Society for Organ Transplantation, ESOT'95; October 3–7, 1995; Vienna, 362.
18. Pielhlmeier W, Bullinger M, Nusser J, et al. Quality of life in type I (insulin dependent) diabetic patients prior to and after pancreas and kidney transplantation in relation to organ function. *Diabetologia.* 1991;34 (suppl I):150–157.
19. Zehrer CL, Gross CR. Quality of life of pancreas transplantation recipients. *Diabetologia.* 1991;34 (suppl 1):145–149.

20. Zehrer CL, Gross CR. Comparison of quality of life between pancreas/kidney and kidney transplant recipients: 1 year follow-up. *Transplant Proc.* 1994;26:508–509.
21. Sutherland DER, Goetz FC, Najarian JS. Living-related donor segmental pancreatectomy for transplantation. *Transplant Proc.* 1994;26:508–509.
22. Hering BJ. Insulin independence following islet transplantation in man—a comparison of different recipient categories. *Int Islet Transplant Regist* 1996;6:5–19.
23. Kaufman DB, Field MJ, Gruber SA, et al. Extended functional survival of murine islet allograft with 15-deoxyspergualin. *Transplant Proc.* 1992;24:1045–1047.
24. Shapiro AMJ, Lakey JRT, Ryan EA, Kozbutt GS, et al. Islet transplantation in seven patients with Type I diabetes mellitus using a glucocorticoid-free immunosuppressive regimen. *N Engl J Med.* 2000;343:230–238.

Pancreatic Cancer—Are There New Treatment Options?

JUERGEN TEPEL and HOLGER KALTHOFF
*Department of General Surgery and Thoracic Surgery, University Hospital of Schleswig-Holstein,
Campus Kiel, Germany*

1.   INTRODUCTION

Nearly 70 years after the first publication of a pancreaticoduodenectomy for pancreatic cancer[1], still only a minority of the patients (10–15%) are candidates for curative resection at diagnosis due to advanced tumor growth[2]. Despite technical advances within the past years, the long-term survival after curative duodenohemipancreatectomy has remained at about 20% in most series[3-8] which is essentially caused by a high rate of local recurrence (up to 70%)[9].

To improve these results there is therefore a persisting need for new (adjuvant or neoadjuvant) treatment protocols employing available modalities and to develop novel therapeutic options based on the growing understanding of the molecular biology of pancreatic cancer.

2.   ADJUVANT THERAPY

As chemoradiation has shown to be efficient in the palliative treatment of unresectable pancreatic cancer and superior to chemotherapy alone, there was hope that this would also contribute to reduce the rate of locoregional failure. After, the Gastrointestinal Tumour Study Group reported a survival benefit for chemoradiation in 1985. Consecutively, these results were confirmed by a number of small series, but in 1999 the large EORTC trial only revealed a trend in favor of adjuvant chemoradiation. Contrary to this, the recently published results of the European Study Group for Pancreatic Cancer (ESPAC)-I trial demonstrated a significant survival benefit for adjuvant chemotherapy (5-FU) but an adverse effect of adjuvant chemoradiation compared to resection alone. Every adjuvant treatment study on pancreatic cancer is impaired by the fact that a significant number of patients do not undergo the planned postoperative treatment due to postoperative complications or patient refusal. Interpretations have therefore to be made carefully. Nevertheless, at present it seems to be likely that survival after curative resection is improved by chemotherapy. Whether gemcitabine is superior to 5-FU is investigated by an ongoing trial (ESPAC-II). Promising results have also been reported from a number of small studies combining external beam radiation therapy (EBRT) with various other substances.

N. A. Habib and R. Canelo (eds.), Liver and Pancreatic Diseases Management, 107–110.
© *2006 Springer. Printed in The Netherlands.*

3.   NEOADJUVANT THERAPY

In theory, there are several advantages to apply chemoradiation prior to resection. A well-oxygenated tissue will be more responsive to radiation, the risk bowel toxicity is decreased as there are usually no fixed loops in the field of irradiation, more patients will actually receive complete treatment, and advanced tumors might even be transformed into respectable ones. Concern was raised whether complications during the chemoradiation might prevent patients from receiving resection, whether the obligatory biliary stenting might increase the complication rate, and whether anastomotic leakage might be more frequent. Meanwhile several reports have shown resection after neoadjuvant chemoradiation to be safe and not associated with an increased morbidity. Anastomotic dehiscence even seems to occur less frequent due to irradiation induced pancreatic fibrosis. Biliary stenting only contributed to an increased rate of wound infections but major complications remained unchanged.

Up to 30% of patients developed distant tumor progression during neoadjuvant chemoradiation and consecutively avoided unnecessary resection. There was some evidence that the site of tumor recurrence was locoregional in only 10% and that 5-year survival exceeded 20%. With growing experience, less patients missed resection of pancreatic tumor due to radiation toxicity but still up to 50% of the patients required hospitalization during chemoradiation. Whether radio-sensitizing agents, which have proved to be efficient in some small trials, will contribute to a substantial improvement of long-term survival remains to be investigated.

4.   NOVEL THERAPEUTIC STRATEGIES

The growing knowledge about the molecular biology of pancreatic neoplasms, with regard to alterations of the genome, proteins, or cellular interaction has led to new targets for tumor therapy. In 2003, 36 of 47 ongoing clinical trials (phase I–III) on pancreatic cancer were testing new anticancer agents (http://cancernet.nci.nih.gov).[10–32]

To enable the growing tumor to infiltrate normal tissue, the so-called metalloproteinases are needed that open up connective tissue and therefore allow tumor cells to penetrate. A specific inhibition of these proteinases could thus reduce its metastatic potential. In fact, Marimastat, a metalloproteinase inhibitor, has shown comparable results to gemcitabine as first line therapy in patients with unresectable pancreatic cancer.

Once the tumor has started to grow, it relies on sufficient blood supply which requires neoangiogenesis. Inhibitors of angiogenesis have been investigated in different tumor entities and have been demonstrated to reduce the metastatic potential of pancreatic cancer in vitro.

A number of genes are either inactivated or abnormally active in pancreatic cancer, such as p53, DPC4, p16, K-ras, and others. Concepts of gene therapy are the reintroduction of inactivated tumor suppressor genes, the increase of susceptibility toward chemotherapy or the increase of immunogenicity. Among different gene delivery systems, which have been tested currently, viral vectors are the most widely used. After some drawbacks, the initial euphoria in gene therapy has been replaced by a more realistic approach. Nevertheless, if safety and efficiency of gene therapy will further improve, it might be a potent therapeutic toll in the future.

The result of mutations in oncogenes can be a so-called gain of function. To inhibit these, pathological gene activity is the object of antisense oligonucleotides that bind to a specific sequence of the mRNA, thus inhibiting their translation into proteins. The efficacy of antisense oligonucleotides directed against p53 has been shown in vivo (Lit). Besides that modified oligonucleotides are capable to inhibit pancreatic tumor growth in different ways as shown in animal experiments (Lit). Other possibilities to alter biological behavior of pancreatic cancer by nucleic acids are siRNA or immune stimulatory, the so-called CpG oligonucleotides which contain cytidyl-guanosyl dinucleotides. The target of immunotherapy is overexpressed proteins such as MUC-1, CEA, and K-ras, which are unfortunately not entirely specific for pancreatic tumor cells. Monoclonal antibodies against these antigens have been tested and despite limited clinical responses in initial studies this approach might play a role in the future. The application of antitumor vaccines consisting of tumor cells, peptides or proteins has been tested with limited success so far. Another vaccination strategy is the extraction of antigen presenting dendritic cells from the patient, which are reapplied after ex vivo loading with tumor-specific antigens. Although this concept has been proved to generate specific effector cells, so far no clinically relevant growth inhibition of tumor has been demonstrated.

REFERENCES

1. Brunschwig A. A one-stage pancreaticoduodenectomy. *Surg Gynecol Obstet.* 1937;65:681–684.
2. Wanebo HJ, Vezeridis MP. Pancreatic carcinoma in perspective. A continuing challenge. *Cancer.* 1996;78(suppl 3):580–591.
3. Lillemoe KD. Current management of pancreatic carcinoma. *Ann Surg.* 1995;221(2):133–148.
4. Ishikawa O. Surgical technique, curability and postoperative quality of life in an extended pancreatectomy for adenocarcinoma of the pancreas. *Hepatogastroenterology.* 1996;43(8):320–325.
5. Richter A, Niedergethmann M, Sturm JW, Lorenz D, Post S, Trede M. Long-term results of partial pancreaticoduodenectomy for ductal adenocarcinoma of the pancreatic head: 25-year experience. *World J Surg.* 2003;27(3):324–329.
6. Henne-Bruns D, Vogel I, Lüttges J, Klöppel G, Ductal KB. Adenocarcinoma of the pancreas head: survival after regional versus extended lymphadenectomy. *Hepatogastroenterology.* 1998;45(21):855–866.
7. Magistrelli P, Antinore A, Crucitti A, La Greca A, Masetti R, Coppola R, Nuzzo G, Picciochi A. Prognostic factors after surgical resection for pancreatic carcinoma. *J Surg Oncol.* 2001;74(1):36–40.
8. Lim JE, Chien MW, Earle CC. Prognostic factors following curative resection for pancreatic adenocarcinoma. *Ann Surg.* 2003;237:74–85.
9. Sperti C, Pasquali C, Piccoli A, Pedrazzoli S. Recurrence after resection for ductal adenocarcinoma of the pancreas. *World J Surg.* 1997;21(2):195–200.
10. Fisher BJ, Perera FE, Kocha W, et al. Analysis of the clinical benefit of 5-fluorouracil and radiation treatment in locally advanced pancreatic cancer. *Int J Radiat Oncol Biol Phys.* 1999;45:291–295.
11. Kalser MH, Ellenberg SS. Pancreatic cancer. Adjuvant combined radiation and chemotherapy following curative resection (published erratum appears in *Arch Surg.* 1986;121:1045) *Arch Surg.* 1985;120:899–903.
12. Whittington R, Bryer MP, Haller DG, et al. Adjuvant therapy of resected adenocarcinoma of the pancreas. *Int J Radiat Oncol Biol Phys.* 1991;21:1137–1143.
13. Foo ML, Gunderson LL, Nagorney DM, et al. Patterns of failure in grossly resected pancreatic ductal adenocarcinoma treated with adjuvant irradiation +/−5 fluorouracil. *Int J Radiat Oncol Biol Phys.* 1993;26:483–489.

14. Yeo CJ, Abrams RA, Grochow LB, et al. Pancreaticoduodenectomy for pancreatic adenocarcinoma: postoperative adjuvant chemoradiation improves survival. A prospective, single institution experience. *Ann Surg.* 1997;225:621–633.
15. Klinkenbijl JH, Jeekel J, Sahmoud T, et al. Adjuvant radiotherapy and 5-fluorouracil after curative resection of cancer of the pancreas and periampullary region: phase III trial of the EORTC gastrointestinal tract cancer cooperative group. *Ann Surg.* 1999;230:776–782.
16. Neoptolemos JP, Stocken D, Friess H, Bassi C, Dunn JA, Hickey H, Beger H, Fernandez-Cruz L, Dervenis C, Lacaine F, Falconi M, Pederzoli P, Pap A, Spooner D, Kerr DJ, Büchler M. A 2004, randomized trial of chemoradiotherapy and chemotherapy after resection of pancreatic cancer. *N Engl J Med.* 1998;350:1200–1210.
17. Nukui Y, Picozzi VJ, Traverso LW. Interferon-based adjuvant chemoradiation therapy improves survival after pancreaticoduodenectomy for pancreatic carcinoma. *Am J Surg.* 2000;179:367–371.
18. Todd KE, Gloor B, Lane JS, et al. Resection of locally advanced pancreatic cancer after downstaging with continuous-infusion 5-fluorouracil, mitomycin-C, leucovorin and dipyrimidamole. *J Gastrointest Surg.* 1998;2:159–166.
19. Chakravarthy A, Abrams RA, Yea CJ, et al. Intensified adjuvant combined modality therapy for resected periampullary adenocarcinoma: acceptable toxicity and suggestion of improved 1-year disease free survival. *Int J Radiat Oncol Biol Phys.* 2000;48:1089–1096.
20. White R, Hurwitz H, Lee C, et al. Neoadjuvant chemoradiation for localized adenocarcinoma of the pancreas. *Ann Surg Oncol.* 2001;8:758–765.
21. Spitz F, Abruzzese J, Lee JE, et al. Preoperative and postoperative chemoradiation strategies in patients treated with pancreaticoduodenectomy for adenocarcinoma of the pancreas. *J Clin Oncol.* 1997;15:928–937.
22. Hoffman JP, Lipsitz S, Pisansky T, et al. Phase II trial of preoperative radiation therapy and chemotherapy for patients with localized, respectable adenocarcinoma of the pancreas: an Eastern Cooperative Oncology Group Study. *J Clin Oncol.* 1998;16:317–323.
23. Ishikawa O, Ohhigashi H, Teshima T, et al. Clinical and histopathological appraisal of preoperative irradiation for adenocarcinoma of the pancreatoduodenal region. *J Surg Oncol.* 1989;40:143–151.
24. Pisters PW, Hudec WA, Hess KR, et al. Effect of decompression on pancreaticoduodenectomy-associated morbidity in 300 consecutive patients. *Ann Surg.* 2001;234:47–55.
25. Pisters PW, Hudec WA, Lee JE, et al. Preoperative chemoradiation for patients with pancreatic cancer: toxicity of endobiliary stents. *J Clin Oncol.* 2000;18:860–867.
26. Breslin TM, Hess KR, Harbison DB, et al. Neoadjuvant chemoradiation for adenocarcinoma of the pancreas: treatment variables and survival duration. *Ann Surg Oncol.* 2001;8:123–132.
27. Pingpank JF, Hoffman JP, Ross EA, et al. Effect of preoperative chemoradiotherapy on surgical margin status of resected adenocarcinoma of the head of the pancreas. *J Gastrointest Surg.* 2001;5:121–130.
28. Wolff RA, Evans DB, Gravel DM, et al. Phase I trial of gemcitabine combined with radiation fro the treatment of locally advanced pancreatic carcinoma. *Clin Cancer Res.* 2001;7:2246–2253.
29. Pisters PWT, Abruzzese JL, Janjan NA, et al. Comparative toxicities of preoperative paclitaxel vs. 5-fluorouracil based rapid fractionation chemoradiation for respectable pancreatic adenocarcinoma. *Proc. Am. Soc. Clin. Oncol.* 1999;18:224.
30. Bramhall SR, Rosemurgy A, Brown PD, et al. Maimastat as first-line therapy for patients with unresectable pancreatic cancer: a randomised trial. *J Clin Oncol.* 2001;19:3447–3455.
31. Fisher WE, Berger DH. Angiogenesis and antiangiogenic strategies in pancreatic cancer. *Int J Gastrointest Cancer.* 2003;33(1):79–88.
32. Von Bernstorff W, Voss M, Freichel S, Schmid A, Vogel I, Johnk C, Henne-Bruns D, Kremer B, Kalthoff H. Systemic and local immunosuppression in pancreatic cancer patients. *Clin Cancer Res.* 2001;7(suppl 3):925s–932s.

Current Practice in Pancreatic Surgery

PHILIPPE BACHELLIER,* JOHN TIERRIS,[#] JEAN C. WEBER,*
and MADHAVA PAI[†]
*Department of Surgery, Centre Hospitalier Hautpierre, Strasbourg, France
[#]Department of Surgery, Hammersmith Hospital, London, UK
[†] Imperial College, London, UK

1.   INTRODUCTION

There are various indications for pancreatic resections but they are essentially destined for treating malignant tumors (solid or cystic), which necessitate a large oncological resection. Endocrine, cystic non-degenerative, intraductal papillary, and mucinous pancreatic tumors (IPMPT) and chronic pancreatitis are equally indications for pancreatectomy. However, under these circumstances a less extensive resection can allow, according to the case, conservation of the pylorus, the duodenum, the spleen, and splenic vessels, permitting at the same time preservation of as much as possible functional pancreatic parenchyma. Traumatic lesions of the pancreas can also, in certain cases, lead to a pancreatic resection. Finally, when curative resection of a malignant pancreatic tumor is found impossible, surgery has still a place in the palliative treatment of the patient, in spite of recent progress in endoscopic and radiologic interventional procedures. In view of this large diversity of pancreatic lesions, resection, when possible, is far more than universal. Existing surgical techniques can be classified into eight categories:

– Pancreatectomies of the head (cephalic)
– Ampullectomies (resections of the ampulla of Vater)
– Left pancreatectomies
– Central pancreatectomies
– Total pancreatoduodenectomy
– Ancillary procedures with pancreatectomies
– Palliative surgical treatment in surgical cancer
– The role of laparoscopy

The surgical treatment of endocrine tumors of the pancreas is not included in this chapter and is examined as a special entity in another chapter.

Resective pancreatic surgery remains a meticulous and demanding operation, requiring special training and skills on the part of the surgeon and long experience in gastrointestinal and also in vascular surgery. In spite of the fact that pancreatic resections for cancer became more complicated with the addition of extensive lymphadenectomies and vascular resections, recent progress in pancreatic surgery has permitted in most centers, a low operative

N. A. Habib and R. Canelo (eds.), Liver and Pancreatic Diseases Management, 111–143.
© 2006 Springer. Printed in The Netherlands.

mortality of less than 3%, although surgical morbidity remains still high, at the level of 20%, due mostly to post-operative pancreatic fistulas.

2.   CEPHALIC PANCREATECTOMIES

The aim of these pancreatectomies is resection of the head of the pancreas. There are many variants of pancreatic head resections, including or not the common bile duct, the duodenum, the stomach, and the jejunum and there are many modalities of reconstruction for re-establishing the biliary, pancreatic, and digestive continuity.

2.1.   Whipple's Operation

Pancreatoduodenectomy (PDC) of the head of the pancreas was first described in 1935 by Whipple, as a two-stage operation, with biliary and gastrointestinal bypass in the first stage and pancreatoduodenal excision effected some days later. Currently, this operation consists of a combined resection of the head of the pancreas, the common bile duct with the gall bladder, the duodenum, part of the distal stomach, and the first centimeters of the jejunum (Fig. 1).

The principal indications of PDC are malignant tumors of the head of the pancreas or the duodenum (pancreatic adenocarcinoma, adenocarcinoma of the ampulla of Vater,

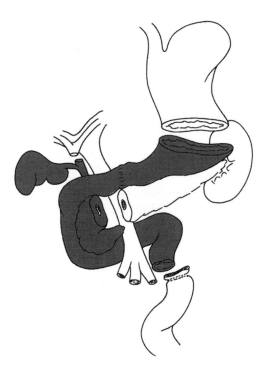

Figure 1. The Whipple operation: resection limits.

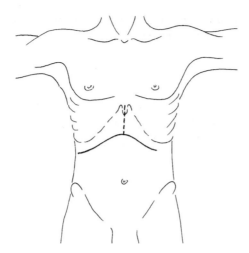

Figure 2. Access to the supramesocolic canal: bilateral subcostal transverse laparotomy ± upper midline extension.

cholangiocarcinoma of the terminal common bile duct, duodenal adenocarcinoma, and cystadenocarcinoma) and pancreatic lesions with degenerative malignant potential, such as localized IPMPT or a mucinous cystadenoma.

Benign lesions of the head of the pancreas are rarely an indication for PDC. A localized chronic pancreatitis simulating pseudo-tumor of the head of the pancreas, even harboring a small malignant focus, in spite of negative intraoperative biopsies and frozen sections, can be a proposed indication for PDC. Furthermore, rare causes of annular pancreas with duodenal stenosis or recurrent pancreatitis can equally represent indications for PDC. Also, the presence of severe derangement of the pancreatoduodenal cephalic complex can lead to a PDC. A bilateral subcostal transverse incision is the most preferred access laparotomy. In case of malignant pancreatic tumor, midline extension of the incision up to the xiphoid process is useful for performing a lymph node clearance (Fig. 2).

As in all pancreatic resections, the operation is following three successive steps: exploration, resection, reconstruction.

2.1.1. Exploration

The purpose of this step is to evaluate the resectability of the tumor, with appreciation of the technical possibilities and the contraindications of resection, such as the presence of peritoneal or liver metastases. The perioperative hepatic ultrasonography can reveal eventful occult metastases.

The exploration is realized following four maneuvers: (1) Opening the lesser sac to the region of the celiac axis and the over-renal aortocaval space. (2) A large coloepiploic separation exposes the isthmus, body, and tail of the pancreas behind the epiploic cavity. (3) The duodenopancreatic dissection (Kocher's maneuver) exposes the aortocaval axis and permits identification of the relationship of the pancreatic head lesion to the celio-mesenteric vascular structures. (4) The cleavage plan between the pancreatic isthmus and the spleno-mesenterico-caval venous axis in order to disclose possible tumor invasion of the veins' wall. During this exposition of the duodenopancreatic block, perioperative pancreatic ultrasonography can help identifying with precision the relationship (possible adherence or invasion) of the tumor to the ductal structures (intrahepatic common bile duct, duct of Wirsung) to the celiac axis, the superior mesenteric artery, and the triple venous axis spleno-mesenterico-portal. The search for celiac–mesenteric arterial anatomic variations (right hepatic artery originating from the superior mesenteric artery, left hepatic artery originating from the left gastric artery, etc.) must be systematic. Failure to identify these variations of the arterial vasculature of the liver can expose to the risk of post-operative is-chemic necrosis of liver parenchyma, in case of ligation of one of these arteries, during PDC. Also, the search for possible stenosis in the origin of the celiac axis from an arcuate ligament must be identified systematically by clamping the gastroduodenal artery. When such a functional stenosis of the celiac axis is present, arterial vascularization of the liver is assured through the gastroduodenal artery, of which the reverse blood flow comes from the superior mesenteric artery through the intermediary of the duodenopancreatic arcade of Rio Branco. The ligation of the gastroduodenal artery, without previous division of the arcuate ligament, results to hepatic arterial ischemia, which can be the origin of lethal, major liver necrosis.

During this exploration phase, biopsy of the pancreatic tumors may confirm malignancy and also lymph nodes from the peripancreatic area, the celiac and aortocaval area are removed and biopsied in order to ascertain the degree of lymph node involvement.

In case of an excretory pancreatic carcinoma with inter-aortocaval lymph node metas-tases, peritoneal carcinomatosis and/or liver metastases, resection by PDC does not improve survival.[5] Under these circumstances, a biliary-digestive bypass is certainly a palliative op-eration less severe than a PDC.

On balance, invasion of neighboring vascular structures and notably of the mesenterico-portal venous axis shows probably a purely local tumor extension and does not constitute a contraindication for resection.[6,7]

2.1.2. Resection

The sequence of events in the operative steps of resection is not constant. The majority of the authors believe that it is more convenient to first liberate the head of the pancreas from its biliary and arterial attachments, divide the stomach before the pancreas for better exposure, and finally divide the jejunum. In our experience, in case of a malignant tumor, we prefer to begin with lymph node clearance of the hepatic pedicle, the retroduodenopancreatic, celiac and inter-aortocaval area. This clearance denudes the vascular structures, completes the exploration, and confirms the possibilities of resection. When the decision to proceed with PDC is taken, the pyloric (right gastric) and gastroduodenal arteries are divided at their origin, respectively, in the proper and common hepatic artery. The common bile duct is divided in the final step of resection and this maneuver avoids leaking of bile into the operative field and unnecessary traction of the portal vein. The division of the stomach is realized at the junction of body and antrum. The division of the jejunum and the liberation of the duodenum are generally effected before dividing the pancreas. During the duodenal dissection, lymph node clearance of the root of the mesentery is also effected, notably at the level of the vascular pedicle of the pancreatic process on the posterior level of the superior mesenteric vascular axis. The pancreas is divided with a scalpel at the level of the pancreatic isthmus, anteriorly to the mesenterico-portal venous axis. A second 0.5 cm piece of tissue is excised from the cut surface of the isthmus pancreas for histology and frozen section. The duodenopancreatic block of the head of the pancreas is further dissected free from the right lateral and posterior surfaces of the mesenterico-portal venous confluence, where tumor infiltration of the retroportal venous wall can be revealed. The discovery, during this stage of resection, of tumor invasion of the mesenerico-portal venous axis, will necessitate a monoblock resection of the infiltrated venous segment. The retroportal part is totally excised in combination with a right splanchnicectomy. Division of the common bile duct, as high as possible, below the proper bile ducts confluence, completes the operation.

2.1.3. Reconstruction

From various reconstruction procedures, the technique of Child described in 1943[8] has become the reference point and remains up to now the "gold standard" of reconstruction. In Child's procedure, the first loop of the jejunum, is successively anastomosed, through the transverse mesocolon, to the pancreatic stump the common bile duct and finally to the gastric stump; a bilateral truncal vagotomy is recommended in order to avoid anastomotic peptic ulcers (Fig. 3).

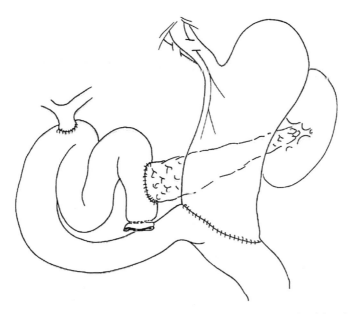

Figure 3. Reconstruction according to Child following PDC: pancreatico-jejunal anastomosis, hepatico-jejunal anastomosis, and anisoperistaltic gastroentero-anastomosis, achieved successively on the first loop of jejunum transmesocolic ± bilateral truncal vagotomy.

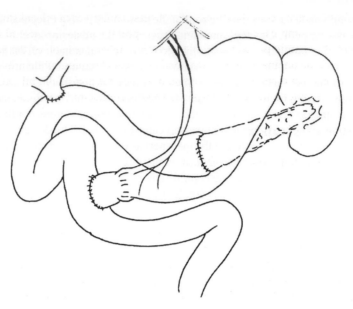

Figure 4. Reconstruction with pylorus preservation following PDC.

3.   VARIATIONS

3.1.   Pylorus Preservation

The PDC of the head of the pancreas with preservation of the pylorus was described by Traverso and Longmire in 1978.[9] This technique is best indicated in the treatment of benign lesions of the head of the pancreas.[10] However, indications for this pylorus preserving procedure have been progressively expanded for malignant lesions, provided they are small in size (diameter < 2 cm) and are located farther from the pylorus.[11] When the pylorus is preserved, vagotomy is not performed. In a classic way, division of the duodenum is accomplished 3–4 cm distant to the pylorus. The pyloric (right gastric) artery must be preferably preserved, in order to secure good vascularization of the duodenal stump, which will be used for the dudeno-jejunal anastomosis (Fig. 4).

This technique of pylorus preservation can be followed by delayed gastric emptying, which can persist for the first two or three post-operative weeks but subsides favorably afterward.

3.2.   Duodenal Preservation

The main indication for cephalo-isthmic pancreatectomies with duodenum preservation using techniques of Beger or Frey and Amikura[12,13] is chronic calcifying pancreatitis invalidating the patient. Furthermore, this type of resection can be utilized in cases of benign lesions, solid or cystic, of the head of the pancreas. As far as chronic pancreatitis is concerned, the operative indication is based on the persistence or recurrence of severe pain, or because of evolutionary complications of the disease (biliary or duodenal stenosis, portal hypertension due to compression of the mesenterico-portal venous axis, pseudocyst formation, etc). Cephalo-isthmic pancreatectomies permit a decompression of the whole ductal pancreatic system, the uncinate process included. These techniques, while preserving more or less healthy pancreatic parenchyma, ascertain decompression of the bile duct, the duct of Wirsung, and the spleno-mesenterico-portal venous confluence.

3.3. Beger's Operation

This procedure includes three steps.

3.3.1. Exposition

The duodenopancreatic head dissection (Kocher's maneuver) permits decompression of the superior genu (first and second part) of the duodenum. In fact, duodenal stenosis due to chronic pancreatitis is generated from adhesions between the duodenum at the level of the superior genu and the retroperitoneal space, formed form the thickened parietal peritoneum from the fibrotic inflammatory process. The superior genu of the duodenum is thus constricted between this fibrous band on top and the hypertrophied head of the pancreas below. Division of this fibrous band during Kocher's maneuver permits ascendance of the duodenum to a higher level, thus eliminating the duodenal stenosis. During this exposition stage, the portal and superior mesenteric vein are dissected above and below the isthmus of the pancreas. The pancreatic isthmus is dissected free from the anterior surface of the mesenterico-portal venous confluence and a sling is passed around it. Also the common hepatic artery is dissected and controlled with another sling at the superior border of the pancreatic isthmus (Fig. 5a).

3.3.2. Subtotal Resection of the Head of the Pancreas

The pancreatic isthmus is divided in line with the mesenterico-portal venous axis. Pancreatectomy of the head and isthmus is further carried out, leaving a residual small portion of the pancreatic head in contact with the inner surface of the duodenum, thus preserving the terminal common bile duct (Fig. 5b,c). On the other hand, the pancreatico-duodenal vascular arcades both anterior and posterior are preserved, with preservation of the gastroduodenal and right gastroepiploic arteries.

After decompression of the intrapancreatic common bile duct, if there is still persisting suprapapillary stenosis of the bile duct, the duct is opened longitudinally in its intrapancreatic trajectory (Fig. 5d). This choledochotomy is kept open by suturing its free edges to the adjacent pancreatic parenchyma and is further included in the pancreatico-jejunal anastomosis that follows.

3.3.3. Reconstruction

Reconstruction with interposed jejunal loop and double pancreatico-jejunal anastomosis. The second jejunal loop is passed through the mesocolon, approximately 30–40 cm

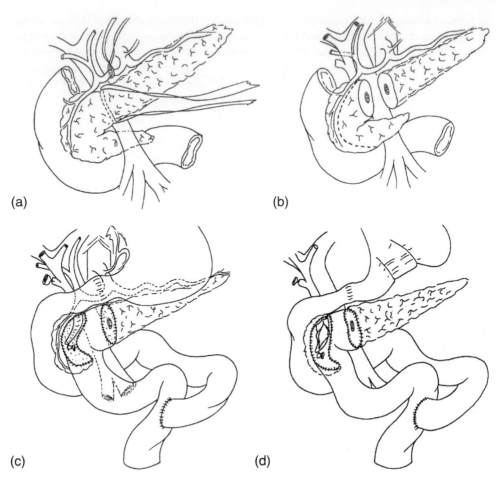

(a)   (b)

(c)   (d)

Figure 5. Beger's operation: (a) Dissection of the pancreatic isthmus, which is surrounded by a sling, control of the common hepatic artery and the origin of the gastroduodenal artery. (b) Margins of cephalo-isthmic pancreatic excision: division of the pancreatic isthmus above the mesenterico-portal venous axis and division of the head of the pancreas inferiorly to the anterior duodenopancreatic vascular arcade with resection of the pancreatic uncinate process. (c) The cephalo-isthmic pancreatic resection leaves in place a slice of head pancreatic tissue comprising the exposed terminal common bile duct. The stump of the Wirsung's duct is ligated. The 2nd jejunal loop is dragged in Roux en Y form over the transverse mesocolon for successive anastomosis to the main pancreatic stump and further to the periphery of the residual pancreatic slice on the inner surface of the duodenum. (d) In case of persisting stenosis of the lower common bile duct following cephalo-isthmic pancreatic resection, the intrapancreatic bile duct is opened with a longitudinal choledochotomy, which is included in the pancreatico-jejunal anastomosis. (e) Longitudinal incision of the duct of Wirsung in the corporeo-caudal pancreatic stump and latero-lateral pancreatico-jejunal anastomosis.

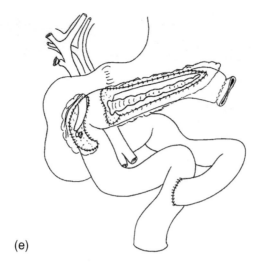

(e)

Figure 5. (Continued)

distal to the ligament of Treitz, in order to be interposed between the two raw surfaces of the remaining portions of the excised pancreas, the cephalic and the body (Fig. 5c,d). The end of this jejunal loop is anastomosed to the raw surface of the residual portion body–tail of the pancreas. This first pancreatico-jejunal anastomosis can be constructed in termino-terminal or termino-lateral manner according to existing or not of a discrepancy in diameter between the jejunal loop and the raw surface of the portion body–tail corporeo-caudal of the pancreas. In case of multiple ductal stenoses of the body–tail corporeo-caudal pancreas, Wirsung's duct is opened longitudinally along the anterior surface of the pancreas, and the ensuing operation is then a latero-lateral pancreatico-jejunal anastomosis (Fig. 5e).

The interposed jejunal loop is afterward anastomosed in latero-lateral way to the raw surface of the remaining pancreatic head. This anastomosis includes the bile duct opening after an eventual suprapapillary choledochotomy (Fig. 5d). Re-establishment of digestive continuity is then secured with a jejuno-jejunal anastomosis at the foot of the loop. Post-operative complications connected to the pancreatico-jejunal anastomoses mostly represented by anastomotic leak and fistula, and digestive bleeding, occur in a percentage of less than 6%. Disappearance of pain in over 80% of patients gives credit to the good quality of the long-term results of this operation.[14]

3.4.   Frey's Operation

This operative technique can be considered as a variant of Beger's procedure. Thus, only the anterior part of the head and the isthmus of the pancreas is removed, with opening of the cephalic part of Wirsung's duct and of the accessory pancreatic ducts (Santorini and ancinar process canal-canal de lincus-). A cephalo-isthmic posterior pancreatic portion of approximately 0.5 cm thick is left in situ. Wirsung's duct of the corporeo-caudal pancreatic stump is opened along its total length by incising the anterior surface of the pancreas (Fig. 6a,b).

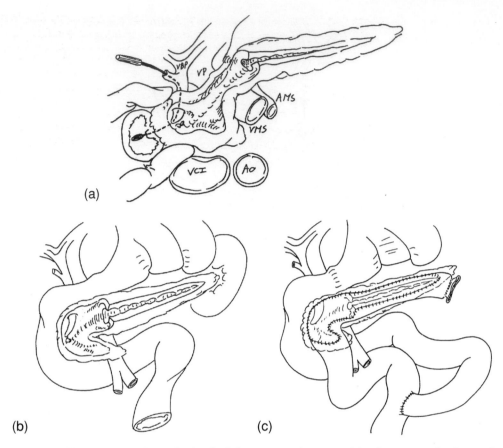

Figure 6. (a) Frey's operation: The head of the pancreas is removed leaving a posterior layer of pancreatic tissue 5 mm thick anteriorly to the mesenterico-portal venous axis. A Bakes dilator can serve to identify the intrapancreatic common bile duct. (b) Incising the Wirsung's duct along the pancreatic body and tail in association with removal of the anterior cephalo-isthmic portion, permits complete exposure of the whole pancreatic ductal system. (c) The jejunal Roux en Y loop is applied over the whole surface of the zone of cephalic pancreatectomy and along the whole length of the corporeo-caudal Wirsungotomy.

   The jejunal loop drawn upward through the transverse mesocolon is anastomosed to the total opening of the Wirsung duct and to the perimeter of the zone of cephalic pancreatectomy, forming in this way a unique pancreatico-jejunal anastomosis (Fig. 6c). As in Beger's technique, the intrapancreatic bile duct is decompressed and in case of a persisting stenosis of the terminal bile duct, a choledochotomy can be done and be included within the pancreatico-jejunal anastomosis in order to secure satisfactory biliary drainage.

   The morbidity and long-term results of this technique do not seem different to those of Beger's technique. However, a prospective randomized clinical study comparing these two techniques showed a 20% morbidity for Beger's operation (pancreatic fistula and gastrointestinal bleeding) and a 9% morbidity for Frey's operation.[15] This study confirmed, however, the good quality of long-term results that were similar in these two groups of patients.

4.   EXTENDED RESECTIONS

Lymph node clearance during pancreatoduodenectomy of the head for malignant lesions of the head of the pancreas. An extensive resection with meticulous lymph node clearance is recommended in the view of improving the results in terms of survival.[16,17] This lymph node clearance comprises the nodes of the hepatic pedicle, the retroduodenopancreatic region, the celiac region up to the inter-aortocaval area superiorly and inferiorly of the left renal vein (Fig. 7a). In this clearance, is also associated a nodal clearance of the root of the mesentery, and of the fibrous, ganglionic, and lymphatic tissue around the origin of the superior mesenteric artery and vein, when the tumor involves the ancinar process of the pancreas and presents with extension to the mesentery (Fig. 7b).

During this extensive lymph node clearance, a complete excision of the retroportal pancreatic portion with right splanchnicectomy is completed, denuding the celio-mesenteric arterial V up to the aorta. Certain Japanese authors combine to the cephalic duodenopancreatectomy with extensive lymph node clearance, a routine resection or the mesentericoportal venous axis.[18] The enlarged resections have sensibly improved the long-term results of cephalic duodenopancreatectomy for cancer and have led above all to diminution of the level of loco-regional tumor recurrence, probably due to the large excision of the splanchnic plexuses. However, destruction of the splanchnic nerves can produce during the post-operative period, acceleration of the bowel transit in the form of hypermotility diarrhea which can, in certain cases, be intractable to medical treatment and invalidate the patient.[19]

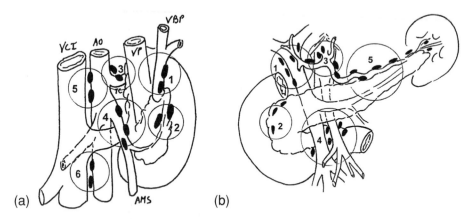

Figure 7. (a) Regional peripancreatic lymph node groups. Posterior view of the duodenopancreatic block: 1 – hepatic pedicle, 2 – retroduodenopancreatic chain, 3 – celiac territory (area), 4 – root of the mesentery, 5 – suprarenal inter-aortocaval territory, 6 – under-renal inter-aortocaval territory. (b) Regional peripancreatic lymph node. Anterior view of the duodenopancreatic block: 1 – hepatic pedicle, 2 – gastroepiploic chain, 3 – celiac territory, 4 – root of the mesentery, 5 – splenic chain.

4.1.   Venous Resection

Invasion of the mesenterico-portal venous confluence from a malignant tumor of the head of the pancreas is no more a contraindication to resection of the head of the pancreas using a cephalic pancreatoduodenectomy.[6] In case of infiltration of the venous wall, excision of the vein must be performed preferably as one piece (monoblock) with the cephalic duodenopancreatectomy operative specimen (Fig. 8a).

The venous excision is represented, according to the site of the venous invasion, by segmental resection of the portal vein, segmental resection of the superior mesenteric vein, or resection of the spleno-mesenterico-portal venous confluence. Reconstruction of the superior porto-mesenteric venous axis is achieved by termino-terminal mesenterico-portal

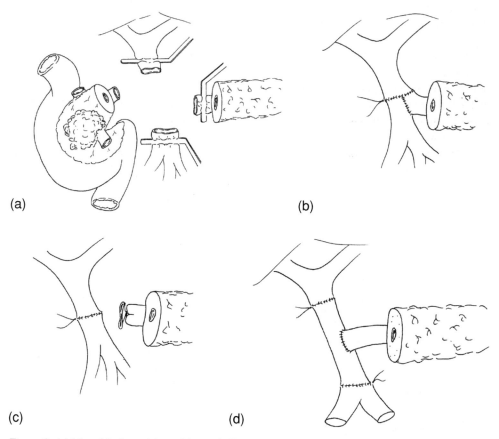

(a)   (b)

(c)   (d)

Figure 8. (a) Monoblock excision of the cephalic duodenopancreatectomy operative specimen and of the spleno-mesenterico-portal venous confluence. (b) Reconstruction of the three-vein axis following PDC with resection of the spleno-mesenterico-portal venous confluence. (c) Termino-terminal mesenterico-portal venous anastomosis with ligation of the splenic vein, following PDC and resection of the spleno-mesenterico-portal confluence. (d) Reconstruction of the spleno-mesenterico-portal venous confluence with vein graft interposition.

anastomosis for segmental venous resections of less than 6 cm in length (Fig. 8b). In case of resection of the spleno-mesenterico-portal venous confluence, reimplantation of the splenic vein is not always mandatory. In fact, when resection of the three-vein axis leaves a long segment of splenic vein, reimplantation of this splenic vein in the mesenterico-portal venous axis can lead, through undue traction, to disturbance of the return splanchnic venous flow. In this case, it is preferable to ligate the splenic vein (Fig. 8c). On the other hand, when resection of the three-vein axis exceeds 6 cm in length in the mesenterico-portal axis, re-establishment of the vascular continuity will be secured by interposition of either a venous graft (internal jugular) or a vascular prosthesis (Fig. 8d).

The mesenterico-portal neoplastic infiltration is an invasion of contiguity, which has no connection to a possible dissemination of the neoplastic disease. The results of PDC of the head of the pancreas with mesenterico-portal venous resection appear to demonstrate an improved survival, which renders this type of excision acceptable, for the additional reason that the post-operative complications do not appear different from those of the standard cephalic PDC.[1,6]

The presence of neoplastic venous invasion can be detected pre-operatively with the help of endoscopic ultrasonography, angiography IRM, or celio-mesenteric angiography, and intraoperative ultrasonography. Nakao et al. has described an angiographic classification, which has demonstrated the importance of venous resection associated to the cephalic PDC when the tumoral stenosis of the mesenterico-portal axis is not complete.[7] On the other hand, when a complete tumoral stenosis is present, associated to a portal cavernoma (stage D of Nakao's classification) despite the technically possible venous resection (excision). There is no gain to be expected in terms of the patient's survival.

4.2. Arterial Resections

During the course of a cephalic PDC, discovery of a tumoral invasion of the common hepatic artery, its right branch or furthermore of a right hepatic artery originating from the superior mesenteric artery, can lead to an arterial resection, in order to obtain a possibly curative resection.[20] Various types of arterial reconstruction can be accomplished, using either a saphenous vein graft, or a vascular prosthesis (Fig. 9a–e). The tumoral invasion of the celiac artery, the celiac trifurcation or more of the origin of the superior mesenteric artery from a tumor of the head of the pancreas, remains in the great majority of cases a contraindication for resection.

4.3. Gastrointestinal (Digestive) Reconstruction

4.3.1. Pancreatic Stump

Pancreatico-jejunal anastomosis In the classic Child's operation, reconstruction following cephalic PDC is (successively) achieved in sequence by pancreatico-jejunal, hepatico-jejunal, and gastroentero-anastomosis. These different anastomoses are carried out using the first jejunal loop drawn upward through the transverse mesocolon. The pancreatico-jejunal anastomosis can be performed in termino-terminal or termino-lateral

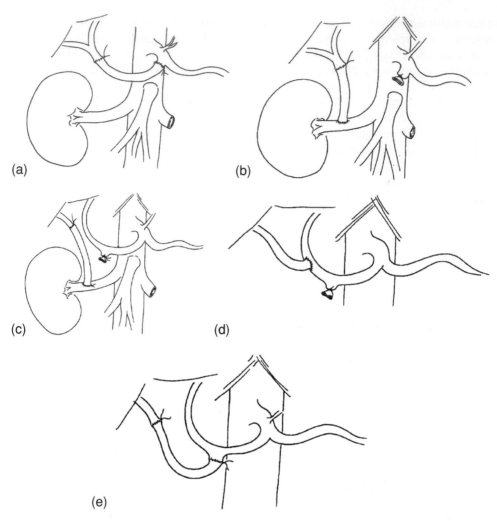

(a)

(b)

(c)

(d)

(e)

Figure 9. (a) Technique of a common hepatic artery reconstruction: saphenous vein graft (or vascular prosthesis) interposed between the celiac trunk and the distal part of the proper hepatic artery. (b) Technique of common hepatic artery reconstruction: saphenous vein graft (or vascular prosthesis) interposed between the right renal artery and the distal part of the proper hepatic artery. (c) Reconstruction of the right branch of hepatic artery or of a right hepatic artery originating from the superior mesenteric artery, using a saphenous vein graft (or vascular prosthesis) interposed and anastomosed to the right renal artery. (d) Reconstruction of the right branch of hepatic artery or of a right hepatic artery originating from the superior mesenteric artery, using a saphenous vein graft (or vascular prosthesis) interposed and anastomosed to the stump of gastroduodenal artery. (e) Reconstruction of a right hepatic artery originating from the superior mesenteric artery by reimplantation to the proper hepatic artery.

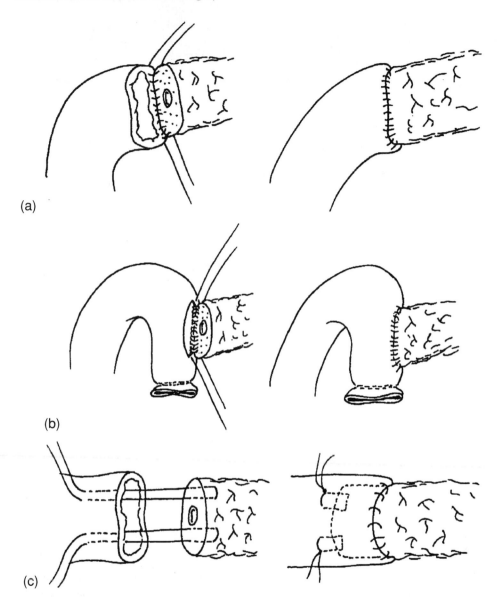

Figure 10. (a) Termino-terminal pancreatico-jejunal anastomosis. (b) Termino-lateral pancreatico-jejunal anastomosis. (c) Pancreatico-jejunal anastomosis by termino-terminal in intussusception (tele-scoping technique) (d) Reconstruction after PDC using a double loop Roux en Y anastomosed, one to the biliary tract and the other to the pancreatic stump.

fashion, depending on the presence or not of disparity between the caliber of the jejunum and the caliber of the pancreatic stump (Fig. 10a,b).

The likelihood of pancreatic leak and fistula following this type of pancreatico-jejunal anastomosis varies from 15% to 35%. According to the sequence of the anastomoses and

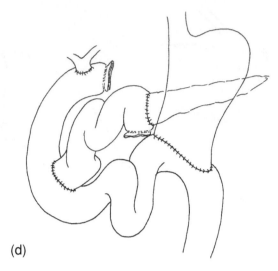

(d)

Figure 10. (Continued)

to the proximity of the hepatico-jejunal anastomosis, a leak (partial rupture) from the pancreatico-jejunal anastomosis can lead to choleperitoneum, which, when there is not sufficient drainage, will require a reoperation. These reoperations after cephalic PDC are followed from a high mortality rate (even higher than 17%) and are generally necessitating a total pancreatectomy.

The termino-terminal pancreatico-jejunal anastomosis by telescoping (telescoping or intussusception technique) has reduced the risk of anastomotic leak and fistula (Fig. 10c). Insertion of a trans-anastomotic drainage tube within Wirsung's duct which is exteriorized (alawitzel) through the jejunal loop can also achieve a reduction in the frequency of pancreatic fistulas in this type of operation.

Furthermore, in order to reduce the risk of pancreatic fistula, the pancreatic anastomosis can be performed to an independent jejunal loop (Fig. 10d).

Pancreatico-gastric anastomosis In order to construct such an anastomosis, the distal gastric resection is more limited. The pancreatic body stump, dissected free from the splenic vein in a distance of 3–4 cm is invaginated into the gastric cavity through a short posterior gastrotomy (Fig. 11a,b).

The anastomosis is completed with interrupted sutures on the perimeter of the gastrotomy (Fig. 11c). In order to avoid bleeding, the gastric mucosa is stitched to the pancreatic capsule with a continuous suture, over the perimeter (periphery) of the pancreatic body stump invaginated into the stomach (Fig. 11d). Some authors perform anastomosis between Wirsung's duct and gastric mucosa over a tube drain.

This type of pancreatic–gastric anastomosis can be equally completed in case of pylorus preservation. In this case, an anterior gastrotomy facilitates invagination of the pancreas

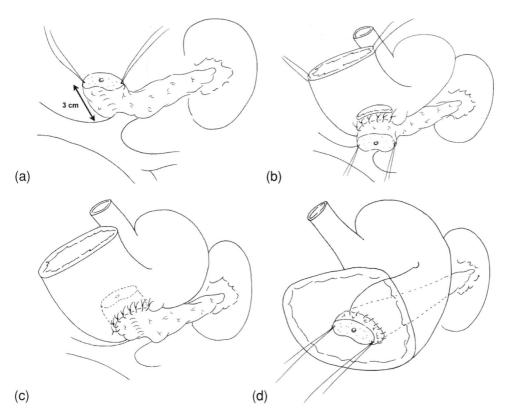

Figure 11. (a) Pancreatico-gastric anastomosis after PDC: dissection free of the pancreatic body stump from the splenic vein. (b) Pancreatico-gastric anastomosis after PDC: mobilization of the body of pancreas toward the posterior surface of the gastric body (anterior plane of the pancreatico-gastric anastomosis) and posterior gastrotomy for invagination of the pancreatic body stump into the stomach. (c) Pancreatico-gastric anastomosis after PDC: invagination of pancreatic body stump within the gastric cavity and sticking of the posterior plane of the pancreatico-gastric anastomosis. (d) Pancreatico-gastric anastomosis after PDC: continuous suture, by endoscopic approach, approximating gastric mucosa to pancreatic capsule over the periphery of the pancreatic body stump invaginated in the stomach.

within the gastric cavity and realization of the pancreatico-gastric anastomosis on the posterior surface of the antrum.

One single prospective randomized study has compared the pancreatico-gastric to pancreatico-jejunal anastomosis. This study has not demonstrated superiority of the pancreatico-gastric anastomosis over the pancreatico-jejunal anastomosis, in terms of pancreatic fistula occurrence.[21] On the other hand, other studies (non-randomized) have disclosed a significant reduction of the frequency of pancreatic fistula ($<$5%) in favor of pancreatico-gastric anastomosis.[22,23] Furthermore, in this case, when this complication

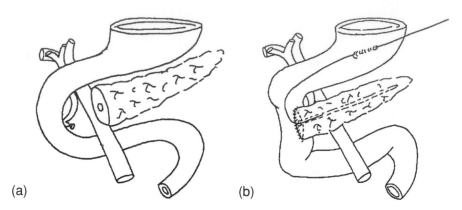

(a)   (b)

Figure 12. (a) Cephalic pancreatectomy with duodenal preservation according to Takada's technique: the head of the pancreas and the uncinar process are resected with conservation of the common bile duct and the duodenum. (b) Cephalic pancreatectomy with duodenal preservation according to Takada's technique: the stump of the pancreatic body is implanted to the interval border of the 2nd part of the duodenum, a pancreatic tube drainage is inserted through the anastomosis and exteriorized in Witzel's way n the anterior surface of the stomach.

occurs, the possibility of gastric aspiration permits a quicker drying of the fistula and significantly avoids reoperations.

Pancreatico-duodenal anastomosis   Takada et al.[24] have reported a small series of true cephalic pancreatectomies leaving no pancreatic tissue on the internal surface of the duodenum (Fig. 12a). The gastroduodenal artery must be preserved in order to conserve the posterior duodenopancreatic arcade which assures the blood supply of the common bile duct. The retroportal pancreatic tissue must equally be preserved. The intrapancreatic bile duct is totally denuded down to the ampulla of Vater. The cephalic duct of Wirsung is ligated and divided at the edge of Vater's ampulla. Re-establishment of the pancreatico-digestive continuity is assured by construction of a pancreatico- or Wirsungo-duodenal anastomosis at the inner border of the second part of the duodenum. This anastomosis is, according to the author's experience, intubated with a tube drain exteriorized on the anterior surface of the stomach (Fig. 12b).

This type of resection exposes to ischemic risk of the duodenum and mostly the duodenal papilla, because of the duodenal denudement during this type of total cephalic pancreatectomy with duodenal preservation.

In the same spirit, another Japanese team has described the isolated resection of the inferior part of the head of the pancreas for localized TIPMP.[25] The totality of the uncinar process and the inferior cephalic pancreas encircling the cephalic part of Wirsung's duct are resected, with conservation of the duodenopancreatic vascular arcades anterior and posterior. The raw surface of the divided pancreas is then anastomosed to the third part of the duodenum in termino-lateral fashion with trans-anastomotic intubation of Wirsung's duct, either with or remaining short tube or with a long tube exteriorized on Witzel's fashion (Fig. 13). This technique has the advantage of preserving the duodenum and also of assuring

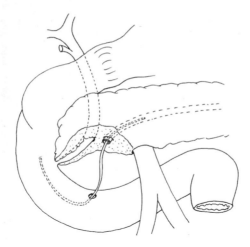

Figure 13. Inferior cephalic pancreatectomy and pancreatico-duodenal anastomosis to the 3rd part of duodenum with a short drain.

the integrity of endocrine and exocrine pancreatic functions. However, the level of pancreatic fistula is increased to the rate of 40%.

4.3.2. The Gastric Stump

Termino-lateral gastro-jejunal anastomosis (Polya type)   This is the gastroentero-anastomosis performed in Child's classic technique. This gastroentero-anastomosis is done in anisoperistaltic way over the whole length of the divided stomach. In order to minimize the risk of post-operative bleeding, it is preferable to fashion this anastomosis in two layers, one mucosa to mucosa and the second extra-mucosal. The anastomosis is placed below the transverse mesocolon.

Gastro-jejunal anastomosis on a Roux en Y loop   In order to avoid biliary reflux into the gastric cavity, it is essential to isolate the gastric stump by the intermediary of a Roux en Y loop anastomosed in termino-lateral fashion to the stomach.

Ampullectomies or resections of the ampulla of Vater   This type of resection is reserved to benign tumors of the ampulla of Vater. In fact, when we are dealing with an adenocarcinoma of the ampulla of Vater or a small periampullary carcinoma (<2 cm), the treatment of choice is PDC of the head with pylorus preservation which enables to respect the criteria of an oncological resection.[26] On the other hand, a benign ampullary tumor can be an indication for local excision. There are two types of excision:

The papillectomy indicated only for mucosal tumors limited to the duodenal papilla (Fig. 14a)

The ampullectomy, which is performed for tumors developing at the lever of the ampulla of Vater (Fig. 14b).

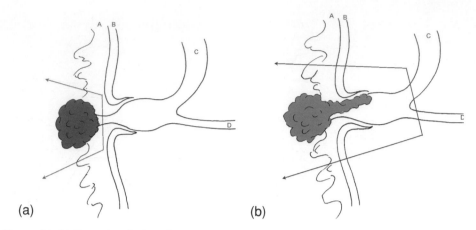

Figure 14. (a) Resection limits of a tumor of the duodenal papilla by papillectomy: A – duodenal mucosa, B – duodenal muscularis mucosa, C – intrapancreatic bile duct, D – duct of Wirsung. (b) Resection limits of Vater's ampulla by ampullectomy: A – duodenal mucosa. B – duodenal muscularis mucosa, C – Intrapancreatic bile duct, D – duct of Wirsung.

During the phase of perioperative exploration, Kocher's maneuver permits palpation of the tumor and removal of retroduodenopancreatic lymph nodes for histological examination (frozen section). In case of discovering metastatic nodes, local excision must be abandoned in favor of a PDC. The same decision must be taken, if palpation or per-operative ultrasonography reveal an ampullary tumor of big size (>2 cm) or a tumoral extension to the depth of periampullary pancreatic parenchyma. For each of the above excisions, approach to the duodenal papilla is achieved through a transverse or longitudinal duodenectomy. The duodenal papilla is located beforehand by transcystic catheterization of the common bile duct, after cholecystectomy, using a Bakes dilator or a "Fogarty" balloon catheter (Fig. 15a). The duodenectomy is kept open using traction sutures. Traction sutures are then inserted round the duodenal papilla.

During the papillectomy the duodenal mucosa is incised in elliptic fashion round the papilla, down to the duodenal muscularis which is saved (Fig. 15b). The submucosal cleavage plane leads to the common channel, which is divided, preferably by scalpel, within the plane of duodenal muscularis without being detached from the duodenal wall. Histological examination (frozen section) of the duodenal papilla verifies that the division goes through healthy tissue and confirms the absence of malignant invasion at the level of the incision near the tumor. In order to complete local hemostasis, the duodenal mucosa can be sutured to the edges of the common channel with interrupted absorbable sutures.

During ampullectomy, the whole Oddi's region is resected, including the periampullary duodenal wall with the zone of the sphincter of Oddi, Vater's ampulla in total as well as a collar of periampullary pancreatic parenchyma. During dissection, the bile duct and the duct of Wirsung are visualized and then divided at supra-ampullary level (Fig. 15c). The excised specimen is first sent for histological examination (frozen section). When excision is found to be incomplete, even in absence of malignancy, and more over when there is an ampullary lesion susceptible to degenerative transformation, the situation will be resolved

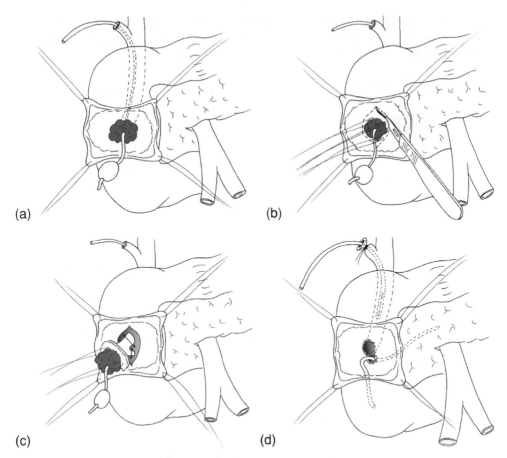

Figure 15. (a) Transduodenal approach of a tumor of the duodenal papilla or of the ampulla of Vater. Location of the papilla using a Fogarty balloon catheter introduced into the common bile duct through the cystic duct, following cholecystectomy. (b) Transduodenal papillectomy or ampullectomy: elliptical incision in the periphery of the duodenal papilla. (c) Ampullectomy: The whole of the ampulla of Vater is incised circumferentially producing a pedicle over the bile duct and Wirsung's duct which are separately divided at supra-ampullary level. (d) Ampullectomy: reimplantation of the common bile duct and the duct of Wirsung reanastomosed in a double canon manner. At the end of those two types of excision, the duodenectomy is closed by duodenal suture. It is preferable to leave in situ an external biliary drainage (transcystic tube drain or a Kehr's tube) which permits decompression of the duodenal suture, but also a post-operative cholangiographic control.

with a cephalic PDC. Following ampullary excision, the bile duct and the duct of Wirsung are found dilated because of the tumoral obstruction. Fusion of the two ducts by lateral suture in double canon fashion will facilitate their duodenal implantation, which is carried out by suture to the duodenal edges with interrupted absorbable stitches (total muscularis-mucosal stitches) on the circumference of the ampullectomy. When, in spite of this, Wirsung's duct is of marrow caliber its drainage can be assured by inserting a fine tube either short (Fig. 15d) or long, exteriorized in Witzel's form.

When the ampullectomy involves a small periampullary collar of healthy and friable pancreatic parenchyma, the risk of post-operative acute pancreatitis can be lowered by duodenal exclusion through a gastro-jejunal anastomosis and bilateral truncal vagotomy.

4.4.   The Left Pancreatectomies (Body–Tail Pancreatectomies)

4.4.1.   Pancreatectomy of the tail (caudal)

The caudal pancreatectomy involves resection of the tail of the pancreas that is of the pancreatic segment to the left of the origin of the superior mesenteric artery. In case of malignant lesion of the tail of the pancreas, the splenic vessels cannot be preserved and the spleen is resected in a monoblock fashion with the tail of the pancreas by caudal splenopancreatectomy. The posterior epiploic cavity is explored after a large coleopiploic separation. The gastro-splenic ligament is ligated and divided. After mobilization of the splenic flexure of the colon, the spleen and the tail of the pancreas are dissected free from the left retroperitoneum till the left border of the root of the mesentery. The splenic artery and vein are ligated and divided at the edge of the pancreatic transaction. This pancreatic transaction is done at the left border of the superior mesenteric artery (Fig. 16a) with a scalpel, with dissection and visualization of the duct of Wirsung by use of the ultrasonic scalper in order to achieve selective ligation of the duct of Wirsung (Fig. 16b). This selective

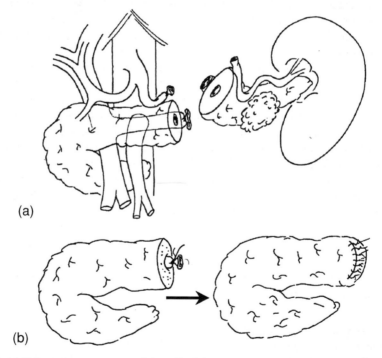

(a)

(b)

Figure 16. (a) Splenopancreatectomy of the tail of the pancreas. (b) Selective ligation of Wirsung's duct and fish-mouth closure of the divided pancreatic surface, following caudal pancreatectomy.

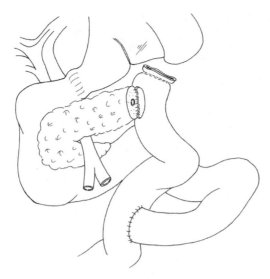

Figure 17. Anastomosis of the transected caudal pancreatic surface to a Roux en Y jejunal loop in termino-lateral fashion after caudal pancreatectomy.

ligation of Wirsung's duct protects against the risk of post-operative pancreatic fistula. The pancreatic stump is then sutured using a fish-mouth technique (Fig. 16b).

When a benign lesion of the tail of the pancreas is present, caudal pancreatectomy can be accomplished with preservation of the splenic vessels.[27] In this case, following approach of the posterior epiploic cavity by coloepiploic dissection, the splenic artery is controlled using a surrounding sling at the edge of the pancreatic transaction. Dissection of the inferior surface of the caudal pancreas permits localization of the splenic vein which is also controlled with a surrounding sling. After transaction of the pancreas at the corporeo-caudal junction, its tail is dissected free of the splenic vessels toward the splenic hilum by ligation of small arterial caudal pancreatic branches, as well as of small draining veins on the anterior surface of the splenic vein. The pancreatic stump is treated in the same manner/way with selective ligation of the duct of Wirsung and closure of the raw pancreatic section in a fish-mouth fashion. The caudal pancreatectomies can also be achieved by laparoscopic surgery. In a case of caudal resection, in the evaluation of a chronic pancreatitis for a pseudocyst with central occlusion of the cephalic or corporeal duct of Wirsung, it is preferable to construct a pancreatico-jejunal anastomosis using a jejunal Roux en Y loop anastomosed termino-laterally to the transected caudal pancreatic surface, in order to obtain goof flow of the pancreatic juice and thus avoid occurrence of a pancreatic fistula on the part of the caudal pancreatic stump (Fig. 17).

4.4.2.   Corporeo-caudal Pancreatectomy

The technique is the same as in caudal pancreatectomy, but this time the pancreatic excision also involves the body of the pancreas situated in the front of the root of the

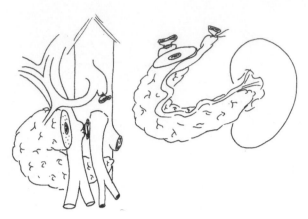

Figure 18. Corporeo-caudal splenopancreatectomy.

mesentery. The transaction of the pancreas is done immediately on the right border of the mesenterico-portal venous axis (Fig. 18). In the same manner, this resection can be accompanied or not by a splenectomy. Keeping in mind the topographic anatomy of the body of the pancreas, a tumoral contiguous invasion, by a malignant tumor of the body, of the celiac trunk, the celiac trifurcation, the origin of the superior mesenteric artery, and the spleno-mesenterico-portal venous confluence is not rare and intervenes in a relatively early stage of the evaluation of the tumor. Discovered through pre-operative morphological explorations, celio-mesenteric vascular invasion by a tumor of the body of the pancreas represents, in general, a contraindication for resection.

4.4.3. Subtotal Pancreatectomy

This type of subtotal pancreatectomy with duodenal preservation, described by Mercadier et al.,[28] preserves a tranche of cephalic pancreas on the duodenal angle (Fig. 19a). The intrapancreatic bile duct is preserved and emerges at the level of the cephalic pancreatic transaction (Fig. 19b). The duodenopancreatic vascular arcades, both anterior and posterior are also preserved.[29]

This pancreatectomy begins regularly from the left with preservation of the splenic vessels, by dissecting free the tail and then the body of the pancreas till the mesenterico-portal venous axis which is uncovered, separated from the head of the pancreas, from the uncinar process (uncus), and also from the inferior part of the pancreatic head. The retroportal tranche of pancreatic tissue is preserved. The intrapancreatic bile duct and the duodenal papilla are located with the use of a Bakes probe introduced beforehand through the cystic duct after cholecystectomy. The common hepatic artery, as well as the gastroduodenal artery are also preserved and the transection of the head of pancreas is effected starting from the superior border of the pancreas, immediately to the left of the gastroduodenal artery, and afterward following a curvilinear trajectory, to a distance of approximately 1 cm from the internal border of the first and second part of the duodenum, until the inferior duodenal angle. The duct of Wirsung, as well as an eventual duct of Santorini, are visualized on the surface of the pancreatic transection and selectively ligated (Fig. 19c).

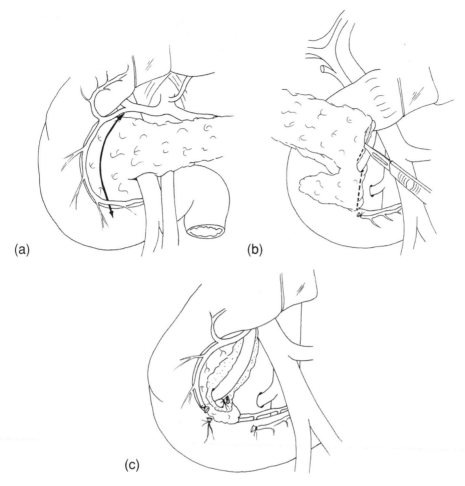

(a)

(b)

(c)

Figure 19. (a) Subtotal pancreatectomy with duodenal preservation: the cephalic pancreatic trans-action (arrow) leaves in place a tranche of tissue from the head of the pancreas on the duodenal angle. (b) Subtotal pancreatectomy with duodenal preservation: the isthmo-corporeo-caudal pancreas is dissected free, from left to right, of the retropancreatic vascular axes, and afterward the cephalic pancreatic transaction is done at the edge of the intrapancreatic bile duct (pointed line). (c) Subtotal pancreatectomy with duodenal preservation: the intrapancreatic bile duct is denuded on the surface of the pancreatic transection which leaves in place a thin piece of tissue from the pancreatic head on the internal surface of the duodenal flexure. The stump of Wirsung's duct is located and ligated over the ampulla.

5.   ASSOCIATED VASCULAR PROCEDURES

5.1.   Appelby's Operation[30]

This operation consists of an isthmo-corporeo-caudal of subtotal pancreatectomy with preservation of the common bile duct, for the malignant tumor of the body or the isthmus of

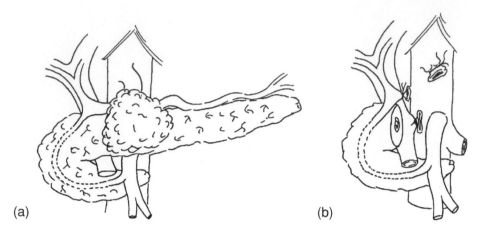

(a)   (b)

Figure 20. (a) Indication of Appleby's operation: corporeal pancreatic tumors invading the celiac trunk and its arterial trifurcation. (b) isthmo-corporeo-caudal splenopancreatectomy with resection of the celiac trunk, the common hepatic artery, the splenic artery, and the left gastric artery.

the pancreas invading the common hepatic artery of the celiac trifurcation (Fig. 20a). In this case, the celiac trunk, the celiac trifurcation and the common hepatic artery are resected in a monoblock fashion with the operative specimen of the left splenopancreatectomy. The blood supply to the liver is assured from the superior mesenteric artery by intermediary of the pancreatico-duodenal arcade and the gastroduodenal artery, which rejoin the middle hepatic artery of the hepatic pedicle (Fig. 20b). In this operation, resection of the mesenterico-portal venous axis can also be associated. The stomach remains vascularized from the gastroduodenal artery by intermediary of the right gastroepiploic and also the pyloric artery.

The blood supply to the liver is preserved through the superior mesenteric artery by intermediary of the pancreatico-duodenal arterial arcade and the gastroduodenal artery.

5.2.   Venous Resections

During a corporeo-caudal left pancreatectomy, an isthmo-corporeo-caudal or subtotal pancreatectomy, resection of the mesenterico-portal venous axis can be associated in case of tumoral invasion. It is then imperative to perform an extensive dissection–separation of the cephalic duodenopancreatic complex according to Kocher's maneuver, in order to secure re-establishment of the venous continuity by termino-terminal free of tension anastomosis, following resection of a venous segment up to 5 or 6 cm in length.

5.3.   The Central Pancreatectomies

The central or median pancreatic resection involves the isthmus as well as part of the whole of the body of the pancreas. Indications for these central pancreatectomies are limited to benign pancreatic lesions or to benign lesions with potential of malignant degeneration: TIPMP localized, serous or mucinous cystadenomas, endocrine tumors.[31–33] Traumatic

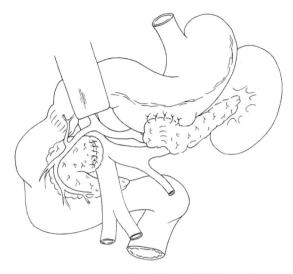

Figure 21. Median pancreatectomy: implantation of the caudal pancreatic stump into the stomach by pancreatico-gastric anastomosis.

ruptures following isthmo-corporeal serious contusion may also require to be treated by central pancreatectomy.[34]

This central pancreatic resection has the advantage of being more economical, in terms of preservation of functional pancreatic parenchyma, than a left pancreatectomy. The distal pancreas must be free of tumoral lesion or of residues of acute pancreatitis. Per-operative pancreatic ultrasonography enables to verify the status of the cephalic pancreatic parenchyma and of the remaining caudal stump. During excision of a central pancreatic tumor, histological examination and frozen section from the right and left transactions is necessary in order to ascertain that they were carried out in a healthy tissue. The splenic vessels are preserved. The cephalic pancreatic stump is closed in a fish-mouth fashion after selective ligation of the duct of Wirsung. The distal pancreas is reconnected to the digestive continuity either by pancreatico-jejunal anastomosis, using a Roux en Y loop, or by a pancreatico-gastric anastomosis (Fig. 21).

5.4.   The Total Duodenopancreatectomy

The principal indications of total duodenopancreatectomy are pancreatic tumors of cephalo-corporeal localization or extending to the near-totality or totality of the pancreatic mass. More rarely, the total duodenopancreatectomy can be performed in presence of a multifocal tumor involving many segments of the pancreatic gland.[35,36]

The intraductal mucinous ectasia (Hai's disease) constitutes an indication for total duodenopancreatectomy.[37] As a matter of fact, the zones of epithelial degeneration can be multifocal or they can involve the whole ductal system of the pancreas. Another reason for performing a total pancreatectomy can appear following a cephalic duodenopancreatectomy, when, in the post-operative phase, a severe complication such as acute pancreatitis or pancreatic fistula on the pancreatic stump occurs. In a same way, an indication of total duodenopancreatectomy can appear during the course of a cephalic duodenopancreatectomy when the tissue of the pancreatic stump is friable and fragile, circumstances that favor occurrence of a pancreatic fistula or of acute post-operative pancreatitis. Concerning the chronic fibro-calcifying pancreatitis invalidating the patient, in patients already operated upon by cephalic duodenopancreatectomy or caudal pancreatectomy, a totalization of the pancreatectomy can exceptionally be carried out when the symptoms persist or evolutionary complications occur. Total pancreatectomy has no more a place in the treatment of acute pancreatitis. The total duodenopancreatectomy can lead to non-negligible secondary sequelae due to the total exocrine pancreatic insufficiency (malabsorption, severe digestion) and to a compete deficit of endocrine secretion (intractable diabetes). These secondary effects (sequelae) that alter considerably the quality of life of the operated patients to a certain extent can be alleviated by preservation of the pylorus.[38] The total duodenopancreatectomy can be completed in two ways (manners): In a monoblock technique, beginning with a large splenopancreatic corporeo-caudal dissection until the anterior surface of the root of the mesentery and notably of the mesenterico-portal venous axis, with the resection continued in the form of cephalic duodenopancreatectomy.[2,3] Or in two steps, when during the course of a cephalic duodenopancreatectomy, after excising the specimen, histology (frozen section) of the isthmo-corporeal pancreatic transection reveals tumoral infiltration arising from the tumor of the head of the pancreas. In this case, totalization of the pancreatectomy, by complementary corporeo-caudal splenopancreatectomy, is performed during the same.[44]

6.   PROCEDURES ASSOCIATED TO PANCREATECTOMY

6.1.   The Splanchnicectomies

The splanchnic plexus is situated in the arterial celio-mesenteric V in the root of the mesentery. During the course of a cephalic duodenopancreatectomy, extensive lymph node clearance associated with excision of the retroportal pancreatic tissue also involves the right splanchnic plexus. In the course of total pancreatectomy, a bilateral surgical splanchnicectomy can be completed in the same manner. When the total of the splanchnic plexus is not resected during the pancreatic excision, a chemical splanchnicectomy with alcohol can be effected as an antalgic maneuver.

6.2.   The Feeding Jejunostomy

Patients suffering from a malignant tumor of the pancreas usually present with an alteration in their general condition and a variable degree of malnutrition. Pre-operative parenteral nutrition can, in extreme cases, be proved necessary.

In order to regain in the shortest possible time an enteral nutrition in these severely undernourished patients, it is preferable to introduce, during the operation, a feeding jejunostomy with its end positioned distal to the gastrointestinal anastomoses. In this way, alimentation can restart right from the 3rd or 4th post-operative day. These jejunostomy tubes can be introduced through naso-esophageal way, pushed through the gastroentero-anastomosis into the efferent loop of the gastric anastomosis to a distance of 30–40 cm. Enteral alimentation can in this way continue until the 7th to 8th post-operative day. When the duration of the use of this type of jejunostomy tube is predicted to be longer, it is preferable to establish a formal jejunostomy or a feeding gastrostomy, which will be of less discomfort for the patient than a naso-esophageal tube.

6.3.   The Pre-operative Bile Drainage

When a malignant lesion of the head of the pancreas is causing obstructive jaundice, the question arises whether or not to establish pre-operatively a biliary drainage. There is still a debate between supporters of a systematic pre-operative biliary drainage in case of jaundice and these who oppose the drainage with the principal argument that the best biliary drainage is the one achieved by surgery. However, an intermediate course attitude can be followed which consists in effecting a pre-operative biliary drainage in high risk patients, old, undernourished, with a high jaundice (bilirubinemia > 300 µmd/l) and also a beginning of renal insufficiency due to renal toxicity of the biliary salts. This biliary drainage can be accomplished endoscopically or in a percutaneous transhepatic way. The regression of cholestasis improves the patient's condition and also permits the establishment of parenteral nutrition.

6.4.   The Palliative Surgical Treatment of Pancreatic Cancer

Approximately 80% of patients with a pancreatic adenocarcinoma cannot benefit from a resection with curative intention, because of the presence of liver metastases, of peritoneal carcinomatosis and/or of a major vascular invasion.[5]

Under these circumstances, the palliative treatment does not improve survival, but has the purpose to provide a maximum of comfort for the patient by elimination of mechanical complications (such as obstructive jaundice, duodenal stenosis, or obstruction) or painful complications and by reduction of morbidity.

The indications of non-surgical treatments, by use of endoscopic or interventional radiologic techniques (biliary endoprostheses, digestive stents, percutaneous splanchnic infiltration with alcohol) reserved initially to patients in very severe general condition, are progressively extended in the great majority of patients declared unresectable by morphological pre-therapeutic examinations. Due to this fact, indications for palliative surgical treatment have been progressively limited to pancreatic tumors of which the unresectability is discovered per-operatively.

7.   SURGICAL TREATMENT OF OBSTRUCTIVE JAUNDICE

Hepatico-jejunal in a Roux en Y loop represent the most efficacious biliary bypass operation. This anastomosis can be completed in termino-lateral fashion after division of the common bile duct or in latero-lateral fashion when division of the bile duct runs the risk of interrupting the whole or part of a portal cavernoma (venous tortuous dilation) secondary to tumoral obstruction of the portal vein, resulting in corollary hepatic ischemia, a source of post-operative mortality in these undernourished patients with a precarious general condition. The advantage of this hepatico-jejunal anastomosis is to place the biliary bypass in a long distance from the tumor, thus avoiding a very early recurrence of jaundice, contrary to a choledocho-duodenal anastomosis. Also realization of this anastomosis to a jejunal loop transposed anteriorly to the transverse colon is further increasing its distance from the tumor. On the other hand, this hepatico-jejunal anastomosis has the disadvantage of been more time consuming and technically more demanding and delicate. The cholecysto-duodenal anastomosis can be done quicker in shorter time, but requires, in order to be functional, permeability of the cystic duct. The proximity of this anastomosis (to the tumor) and to the cystic duct does not permit a biliary bypass of long duration. Also, if the patient is in need of a quick and efficacious operation, it is preferable to replace the surgical bypass by insertion (pre- or post-operatively) of a biliary endoprosthesis.

8.   THE DUODENAL STENOSIS

The gastrointestinal "stents" introduced endoscopically can still pose problems of obstruction (alimentary or tumoral) and of gastrointestinal bleeding. Their indications are consequently less extensive than those of biliary prostheses. For this reason, the surgical digestive bypass keeps its place in the palliative treatment of carcinoma of the pancreas. This gastroentero-anastomosis is carried out in isoperistaltic way to the posterior surface of the stomach, in its lowest point, but also as long as possible from the pancreatic tumor. In order to comply with the greatest possible distance from the tumor, the gastroentero-anastomosis which is usually transmesocolic, can be accomplished in a pre-colic way, particularly when one is dealing with a corporeo-caudal tumor. The first loop of the jejunum is preferably used as an excluded loop (Roux en Y), and the anastomosis is performed in latero-lateral fashion, approximately 20 cm distally to the angle of Treitz. When a biliary bypass by hepatico-jejunal anastomosis is associated to a gastroentero-anastomosis, the anastomosis of the foot of the loop (distal) is constructed on the first jejunal loop, about 30 cm distally to the gastroentero-anastomosis (Fig. 22).

In the absence of duodenal stenosis, there is no general agreement about the necessity of performing a routine digestive diversion.[39] In the evolution course of unresectable pancreatic carcinomas this complication does not supervene in more than 10–25% of the cases.[40,41] However, addition of a gastroentero-anastomosis to the surgical biliary diversion does not increase post-operative morbidity compared to bilio-digestive diversion alone.[42,43] In our experience, when non-resectability of the pancreatic tumor is discovered during the operation, a gastroentero-anastomosis is systematically associated to the bilio-digestive division, the latest being preferably a hepatico-jejunal anastomosis. It is preferable not to add a bitruncular vagotomy in order to avoid gastropexy and post-operative diarrhea, because the risk of developing a peptic (anastomotic) ulcer is minimal in these patients with short life expectancy. On the other hand, if non-resectability is confirmed pre-operatively, in case of obstructive jaundice without duodenal stenosis, the patient can benefit if applying non-surgical treatment by biliary prosthesis introduced through endoscopic or percutaneous transhepatic way.

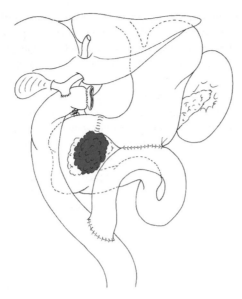

Figure 22. Double biliary and digestive palliative bypass by hepatic-jejunal anastomosis and isoperistaltic gastroentero-anastomosis for unresectable pancreatic tumor.

In all cases of palliative surgical intervention, a splanchnic alcohol infiltration as an antalgic maneuver completes the biliary and digestive diversion.

9.   THE PLACE OF LAPAROSCOPY

With the exception of some PDC achieved in anecdotal way,[4] the pancreatic resections effectuated by laparoscopy are limited to caudal pancreatectomies, with or without preservation of the splenic vessels, and to enucleation of the tumors. In all cases the indications are benign pancreatic tumors, but they also include the endocrine tumors.[45–47] Under laparoscopy, drainage of pseudocysts of the pancreas by cysto-jejunostomy or cysto-gastrostomy can also be achieved.[46] The laparoscopic resection techniques reproduce in every point the ones executed in formal laparotomy. In malignant conditions, the initial laparoscopy performed immediately before laparotomy and assisted by laparoscopic ultrasonography, permits obtaining additional information on respectability, or rather on non-resectability of the pancreatic tumor.[48] In case of contraindication for resection, a gastroentero-anastomosis can be executed under laparoscopy, associated, in case of obstructive jaundice, to a cholecysto-jejunal anastomosis.[49,50] Another option consists in performing the gastroentero-anastomosis under laparoscopy, followed, in case of obstructive jaundice, by post-operative introduction of a biliary prosthesis. The potentially simpler and of better quality post-operative results of this laparoscopic surgery represent an advantage in patients with a limited life expectancy. However, the risk exists of under-evaluating the possibilities of excision, notably of the mesenterico-portal venous axis, and thus perform a palliative maneuver for a resectable pancreatic tumor.

REFERENCES

1. Schäfer M, Müllhaupt B, Clavien PA. Evidence-based pancreatic head resection for pancreatic cancer and chronic pancreatitis. *Ann Surg.* 2002;236:137–148.
2. Cameron JL, Pitt HA, Yeo CJ, et al. One hundred and forty-five consecutive pancreaticoduodenectomies without mortality. *Ann Surg.* 1993;217:430–438.
3. Trede M, Schwall G, Saeger HD. Survival after pancreato-duodenectomy – 118 consecutive resections without an operative mortality. *Ann Surg.* 1990;211:447–458.
4. Whipple AO, Persons WB, Mullins CR. Treatment of carcinoma of the ampulla of Vater. *Ann Surg.* 1935;102:763–779.
5. Baumel H, Huguier M. Le cancer du pancréas exocrine. Diagnostic et traitement. Rapport présenté au: 93ème congrès Français de Chirurgie (1991) Paris: Springer Verlag, 1991, 1–186.
6. Bachellier Ph, Nakano H, Oussoultzoglou E, et al. Is pancreatectomy with mesenterico-portal venous resection safe and worthwhile? *Am J Surg.* 2001;182:120–129.
7. Nakao A, Harada A, Nonami T, et al. Clinical significance of portal invasion by pancreatic head carcinoma. *Surgery.* 1995;117:50–55.
8. Child CG. Pancreatico-jejunostomy and other problems associated with the surgical management of carcinoma involving the head of pancreas. *Ann Surg.* 1944;119:845–891.
9. Traverso JW, Longmire WP. Preservation of the pylorus in pancreatico-duodenectomy. *Surg Gynecol Obstet.* 1978;146:959–962.
10. Jimenez RE, Del-Castillo CF, Rattner DW, et al. Outcome of pancreaticoduodenectomy with pylorus preservation or with antrectomy in the treatment of chronic pancreatitis. *Ann Surg.* 2000;231:293–300.
11. Mosca F, Giulianotti PC, Balestracci T, et al. Long term survival in pancreatic cancer: pylorus preserving versus Whipple pancreaticoduodenectomy. *Surgery.* 1997;122:553–566.
12. Beger HG, Krautzberger W, Bittner R, et al. Duodenum-preserving resection of the head of the pancreas in patients with severe chronic pancreatitis. *Surgery.* 1985;97:467–473.
13. Frey CF, Amikura K. Local resection of the head of the pancreas combined with longitudinal pancreatico-jejunostomy in the management of patients with chronic pancreatitis. *Ann Surg.* 1994;220:492–507.
14. Beger HG, Schlosser W, Friess HM, et al. Duodenum-preserving head resection in chronic pancreatitis changes the natural course of the disease. A single center 26 year experience. *Ann Surg.* 1999;230:512–523.
15. Izbicki JR, Bloechle C, Knoefel WT, et al. Duodenum-preserving resection of the head of the pancreas in chronic pancreatitis. A prospective, randomized trial. *Ann Surg.* 1995;221:350–358.
16. Henne-Bruns D, Vogel I, Lüttges J, et al. Ductal adenocarcinoma of the pancreas head: survival after regional versus extended lymphadenectomy. *HepatoGastroenterology.* 1998;45:855–866.
17. Imaizumi T, Hanyu F, Harada N, et al. Extended radical Whipple resection for cancer of the pancreatic head: operative procedure and results. *Dig Surg.* 1998;15:299–307.
18. Nagakawa T, Komishi I, Ueno K, et al. Extended radical pancreatectomy for carcinoma of the head of the pancreas. *Hepatogastroenterology.* 1998;45:849–854.
19. Ishikawa O. Surgical technique, curability and post-operative quality of life in an extended pancreatectomy for adenocarcinoma of the pancreas. *Hepatogastroenterology.* 1996;43:320–325.
20. Nakano H, Bachellier P, Weber JC, et al. Arterial and vena caval resections combined with pancreaticoduodenectomy in highly selected patients with periampullary malignancies. *Hepatogastroenterology.* 2002;49:258–262.
21. Yeo CJ, Cameron JL, Maher MM, et al. A prospective randomized trial of pancreatogastrostomy versus pancreatico-jejunostomy after pancreaticoduodenectomy. *Ann Surg.* 1995;222:580–592.
22. Arnaud JP, Tuech JJ, Cervi C. Pancreaticogastrostomy compared with pancreaticojejunostomy after pancreaticoduodenectomy. *Eur J Surg.* 1999;165:357–362.
23. Takano S, Ito Y, Yokoyama T, et al. Pancreaticojejunostomy versus pancreaticogastrostomy in reconstruction following pancreaticoduodenectomy. *Br J Surg.* 2000;87:423–427.
24. Takada T, Yasuda H, Uchiyama K, et al. Duodenum-preserving pancreato-duodenostomy. A new technique for complete excision of the head of the pancreas with preservation of biliary and alimentary integrity. *Hepatogastroenterology.* 1993;40:356–359.

25. Nakagohri T, Kenmochi T, Kainuma O, et al. Inferior head resection of the pancreas for intraductal papillary mucinous tumors. *Am J Surg.* 2000;179:482–484.
26. Chareton B, Coiffic J, Landen S, et al. Diagnosis and therapy for ampullary tumors: 63 cases. *World J Surg.* 1996;20:707–712.
27. Kimura W, Inoue T, Futakawa N, et al. Spleen preserving distal pancreatectomy with conservation of the splenic artery and vein. *Surgery.* 1996;120:885–890.
28. Mercadier M, Clot JP, Melliere D, et al. Technique des duodénopancréatectomies céphaliques. *Ann Chir.* 1967;21:672–676.
29. Kimura W, Muto T, Makuuchi M, et al. Subtotal resection of the head of the pancreas preserving duodenum and vessels of pancreatic arcade. *Hepatogastroenterology.* 1996;43:1438–1441.
30. Furukawa H, Hiratsuka M, Iwanaga T. Extended surgery: left upper abdominal exenteration plus Appleby's method for type 4 gastric carcinoma. *Ann Surg Oncol.* 1997;4:209–214.
31. Sauvanet A, Partensky C, Sastre B, et al. Medial pancreatectomy: a multi-institutional retrospective study of 53 patients by the French Pancreas Club. *Surgery.* 2002;132:836–843.
32. Falconi M, Salvia R, Bassi C, et al. Clinicopathological features and treatment of intraductal papillary mucinous tumour of the pancréas. *Br J Surg.* 2001;88:376–381.
33. Partensky C, Berger F, Ponchon T, et al. Pancréatectomie pour tumeur intracanalaire papillaire mucineuse du pancréas. *Gastroenterol Clin Biol.* 1996;20:938–945.
34. Than LN, Duchman JC, Thon That B, et al. Conservation du pancréas gauche dans les ruptures de l'isthme pancréatique: à propos de 3 cas. *Chirurgie.* 1999;124:165–170.
35. Ihse I, Anderson H, Andren-Sandberg A. Total pancreatectomy for cancer of the pancreas: is it appropriate? *World J Surg.* 1996;20:288–294.
36. Blanchet MC, Andreel F, Scoazec JY, et al. Pancréatectomie totale pour tumeur mucineuse du pancréas. *Ann Chir.* 2002;127:439–448.
37. Kimura W, Sasahira N, Yoshikawa T, et al. Duct-ectatic type of mucin producing tumor of the pancreas – new concept of pancreatic neoplasia. *Hepatogastroenterology.* 1996;43:692–709.
38. Sugiyama M, Atomi Y. Pylorus-preserving total pancreatectomy for pancreatic cancer. *World J Surg.* 2000;24:66–71.
39. Dobermeck RL, Berndt GA. Delayed gastric emptying after palliative gastrojejunostomy for carcinoma of the pancreas. *Arch Surg.* 1987;122:827–829.
40. Baumet H, Huguier M, Manderscheid JC, et al. Results of resection for cancer of the exocrine pancreas: a study from the French Association of Surgery. *Br J Surg.* 1994;81:102–107.
41. Potts JR, Broughan T, Hermann RE. Palliative operations for pancreatic surgery. *Am J Surg.* 1990;159:72–78.
42. Sarr MG, Cameron JL. Surgical palliation of unresectable carcinoma of the pancreas. *World J Surg.* 1984;8:906–918.
43. Singh SM, Longmire WP, Reber HA. Surgical palliation for pancreatic cancer: the UCLA experience. *Ann Surg.* 1990;212:132–139.
44. Gagner M, Pomp A. Laparoscopic pylorus-preserving pancreaticoduodenectomy. *Surg Endosc.* 1994;8:408–410.
45. Fernandez-Cruz L, Saenz A, Astudillo E, et al. Outcome of laparoscopic pancreatic surgery: endocrine and non-endocrine tumors. *World J Surg.* 2002;26:1057–1065.
46. Park AE, Heniford T. Therapeutic laparoscopy of the pancreas. *Ann Surg.* 2002;236:149–158.
47. Patterson EJ, Gagner M, Salky B, et al. Laparoscopic pancreatic resection: single-institution experience of 19 patients. *J Am Coll Surg.* 2001;193:281–287.
48. Nieveen van Dijkum EJM, Romijn MG, Terwee CB, et al. Laparoscopic staging and subsequent palliation in patients with peripancreatic carcinoma. *Ann Surg.* 2003;237:66–73.
49. Shimi S, Banting S, Cuchieri A. Laparoscopy in the management of pancreatic cancer: endoscopic cholecystojejunostomy for advanced disease. *Br J Surg.* 1992;79:317–319.
50. Mouiel J, Kathkouda N, White S, et al. Endolaparoscopic palliation of pancreatic cancer. *Surg Laparosc Endosc.* 1992;2:241–243.